Riddles, Rhyme & Alliteration

Listening Exercises Based on Phonics

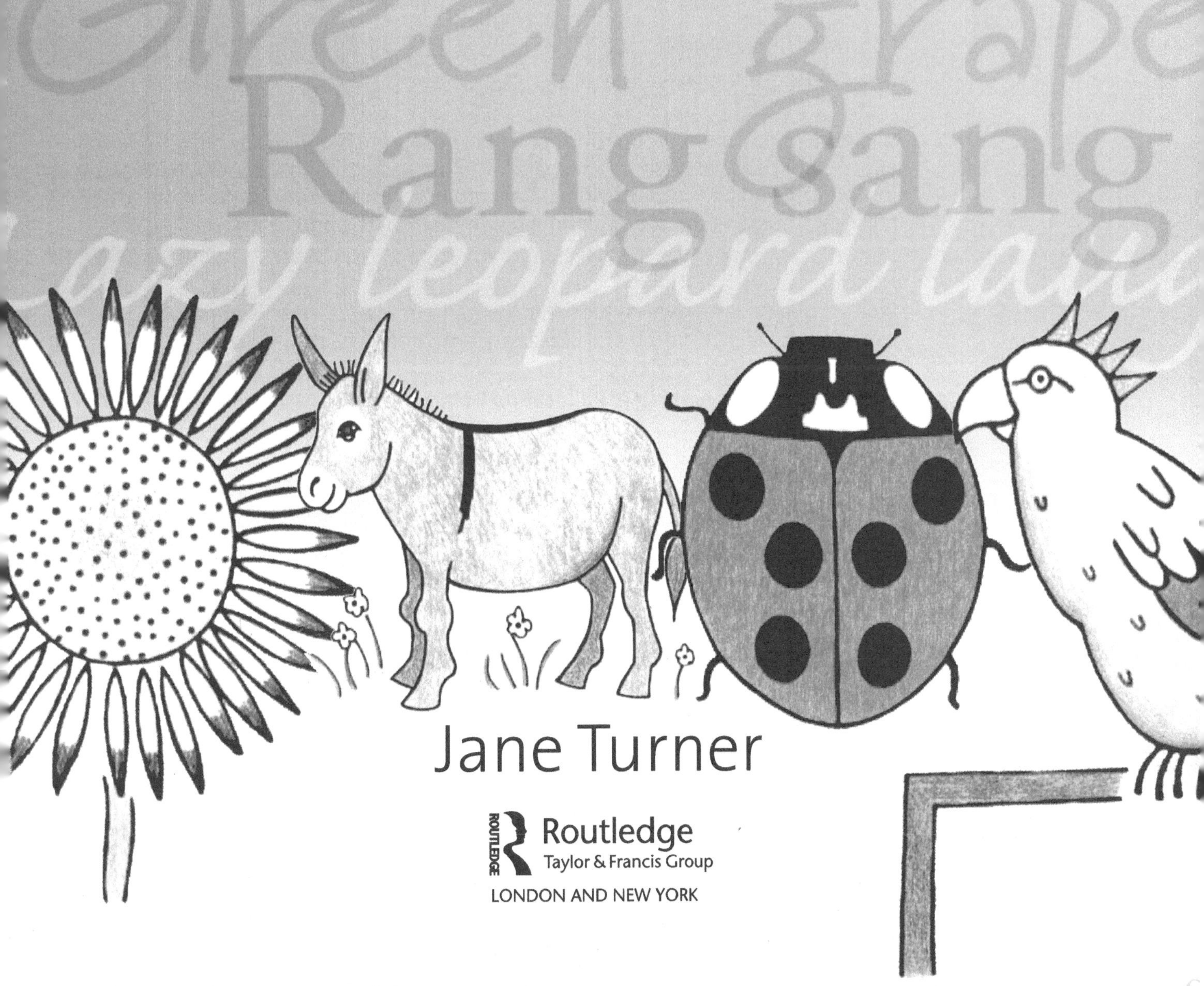

Jane Turner

Routledge
Taylor & Francis Group

LONDON AND NEW YORK

For readers outside the UK, the age ranges for the classes mentioned are as follows: Reception (Year R): 4–5 years and Key Stage 1: 5–7 years. Key Stage 1 is divided into two years, Year 1: 5–6 years and Year 2: 6–7 years. Year 3 (7–8 years) is part of Key Stage 2.

First published 2007 by Speechmark Publishing Ltd.

Published 2019 by Routledge
2 Park Square, Milton Park, Abingdon, Oxon OX14 4RN
52 Vanderbilt Avenue, New York, NY 10017

Routledge is an imprint of the Taylor & Francis Group, an informa business

British Library Cataloguing in Publication Data
Turner, Jane
   Riddles, rhyme & alliteration : listening exercises based on phonics
   1. Hearing impaired children – Education   2. English language – Phonetics –
   Problems, exercises, etc.   3. Listening – Problems, exercises, etc.
   I. Title
   371.9'12

ISBN 978-0-86388-600-3 (pbk)

Contents

Preface

This book contains activities to encourage children to listen, concentrate and consolidate their knowledge of phonics. The activities are aimed at children aged 4–7 (Years R, 1 and 2) but they can also be used with older children who need to develop their ability to listen and/or require more encouragement to master phonic skills.

As an experienced, qualified teacher of the deaf, I have found the 'riddles' activities to be very useful when teaching children who have a language delay and/or a poor vocabulary. I have also used the stories and tongue twisters contained in this book as practice material when teaching adults to become proficient in Cued Speech (a system using lip-reading and hand signals, which is phonetically based and used to teach spoken English to deaf children).

Riddles, Rhyme & Alliteration:

→ Contains various phonemically based activities

→ Requires no extra materials

→ Has clear instructions

→ Can be used alongside any phonics programme

→ Can be used to enhance children's listening skills

→ Is a useful resource for busy teachers.

Introduction

Phonics have, for a number of years, been fundamental to the teaching of reading. 'Synthetic Phonics' programmes already exist, and it is now recommended that all children starting in the reception year (Year R, 4–5 years) should be taught 'Synthetic Phonics' as part of their reading curriculum. It is vital, therefore, that children should be able to concentrate, listen and discriminate between the different speech sounds.

Not all children enter school equipped to cope with learning the phonemes of the English Language. Some may not have developed their listening skills sufficiently, some may have language difficulties that impede upon their ability to process speech sounds, and others may have 'glue ear' or auditory processing problems. The activities in this book are designed to assist these children in improving their listening and sound discrimination abilities. The activities can also be used as supplementary material for any phonics programme. Each activity can be used with individuals, groups or whole classes. The activities are varied and would most suit children in Years R, 1 and 2.

There are 18 sections in this book, which cover the phonemes 'b', 'c/k', 'd', 'f', 'g', 'h', 'j', 'l', 'm', 'n', 'p', 'r', 's', 't', 'v', 'w', 'y', 'th' (unvoiced), 'sh' and 'ch'. Each section has eight different activities, and includes two or three pages of illustrations. The activities are:

→ Riddles, which can be solved with the help of the picture pages
→ An alliteration activity
→ Tongue twisters for the children to repeat
→ An 'Odd word out' activity involving listening for the word that does not begin with the target phoneme
→ An 'Odd word out' activity involving listening for the word that does not rhyme with the other two

→ 'Words to sound out', involving the teacher sounding out the individual phonemes of a word and the children saying what the word is
→ A story that contains words beginning with the target phoneme
→ A 'Puzzle worksheet' based on the words illustrated on the picture pages in the section.

All of these activities are described in more detail in 'How to use this book'.

It is not intended that all the activities in every section should be used with the class, group or individual. The teacher needs to look at the activities in this book and assess which ones will best suit the needs of the children. The riddles activities can be used alone as a vocabulary building or a listening exercise, as explained on page 3. The more phonically based activities can be used as listening exercises or as supplementary material for the phonics scheme used by the class teacher. As all the activities, except the puzzle worksheet pages, are presented orally by the teacher, there is no prerequisite for the children to be able to read any of the written material in the first seven activities of each section.

How to use this book

There are 18 sections in this book, which cover the phonemes 'b', 'c/k', 'd', 'f', 'g', 'h', 'j', 'l', 'm', 'n', 'p', 'r', 's', 't', 'v', 'w', 'y', 'th'(unvoiced), 'sh' and 'ch'. Each section has eight different activities.

For ease of use, instructions for carrying out these activities appear with the activities themselves. Answers for the stories and the puzzle worksheets can be found in a separate section at the end of the book.

Riddles (with illustrations)

This activity consists of 12 riddles based on the target phoneme. There are illustrations, for the children's reference, to accompany the riddles. There are more pictures than there are riddles as the other pictures on these pages are distractors.

The riddles can be used:
→ To teach vocabulary to children who have a language delay, or have English as their second language
→ Alongside a phonics programme to reinforce the target sound
→ For encouraging the children to listen more attentively.

This activity is suitable for children in Year R or for older children if they are experiencing language difficulties or problems with learning phonics.

Alliteration

This activity consists of 12 two-word phrases. All of the phrases include words beginning with the target sound, although in some phrases both words begin with that sound. The aim is for the children to listen for the target sound in the initial position and discriminate between that and other initial sounds.

Tongue twisters

There are five of these in each section. These are sentences that are made up mainly of words beginning with the target sound. The tongue twisters:
→ Help children to develop their auditory memory
→ Help children to listen carefully
→ Draw children's attention to the target sound.

Odd word out — initial sounds

This activity consists of 15 sets of three words each. Two words in each set begin with the target sound, whereas the third does not. The aim is for the children to be able to distinguish between words that begin with the target sound and ones that do not.

Odd word out — rhyming

This activity consists of 10 sets of words. In each set there are two words that rhyme and one that does not. Recognition of rhyming words is part of the Literacy National Curriculum, and having knowledge of rhyming words helps children to learn spelling patterns.

Words to sound out

In each section there are eight words to 'sound out'. Part of the National Curriculum of England and Wales, and a component of the 'Synthetic Phonics' programmes, involves saying each phoneme in a word consecutively and then blending them together to make a word. This activity aims to enable children to blend phonemes together to make words.

> This activity is suitable for some Year R children and those in Years 1 and 2 or above if this skill has not developed sufficiently.

Story

Each section provides a story containing many words beginning with the target sound. The aim of these stories is to:
→ Enhance the children's ability to listen
→ Extend the children's auditory memory
→ To further the children's ability to recognise the target sound in an initial position.
Answers to the story for each section can be found at the end of the book.

> Some Year R children may be able to cope with this, but this activity is more suited to Years 1 and 2 and older children who need more practice in listening skills and/or recognising target sounds in the initial position.

Puzzle worksheet

Each section of this book has a worksheet for children to complete. This worksheet involves two 'puzzles' based on the words that are illustrated as part of the riddles activity. In each section the worksheet has exactly the same format so that when the children become familiar with this, they can try to do the puzzles by themselves. The first task on the worksheet is to look at five words that have each been jumbled up; the children unscramble the letters to make words. The second task is to find eight words in a wordsearch. All the words in both tasks can be found on the picture pages that accompany each section. Answers to the puzzles for each section can be found at the end of the book.

Instructions for the puzzle worksheets

→ The teacher reads and explains the first task to the children, and then the teacher shows the children the worksheet and the picture pages. The teacher proceeds to explain the task, writes the first anagram on the board and suggests that the children look at the words printed under the pictures, to find one which has the same letters as the anagram. Then the teacher invites a child to write the correct word on the board. When two or three examples have been completed, the children can try and finish this part of the worksheet on their own.

→ If the classroom has an interactive whiteboard, the worksheet could be scanned into the computer, and the teacher could then proceed as above. The teacher should point out as they go along that the words used in this activity can be found on the picture sheets.

→ The teacher reads the instructions on the page for the wordsearch and explains the task. If the teacher does this on each occasion for the first two or three worksheets, the children can try to complete the next ones by themselves without being shown any examples.

→ If the children are more capable, the teacher gives out the worksheets and the pictures as mentioned above, and goes through the instructions with the children. They then try to complete the tasks by themselves. Children who are more capable can try and do the tasks without reference to the pictures.

This activity is more suitable for Years 1 and 2. Some Year R children may be able to do the tasks on the worksheet towards the end of that academic year, and these worksheets may also be suitable for some Year 3 children who are experiencing difficulties with reading skills.

Section for the 'b' sound

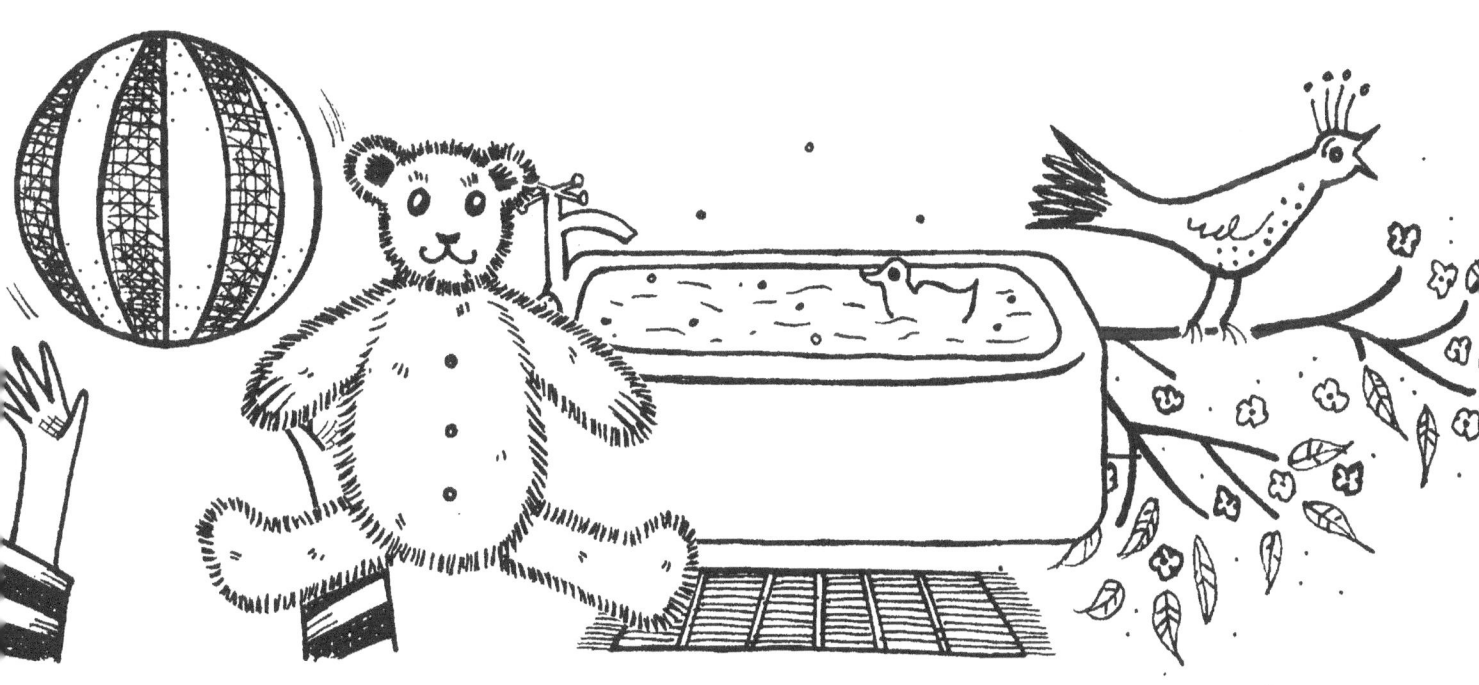

Section for the 'b' sound

Riddles for the 'b' sound

→ Children are given the photocopied pictures to go with the target sound. The teacher reads out the riddles, one at a time, and the children decide which picture each one refers to. If desired, the children can then colour these pictures in.

→ *To make the activity more difficult*, the children, without access to the pictures, are told the target sound, and the riddles are read out one at a time. The children have to think of something that starts with that sound and fits in with the riddle.

→ *To teach vocabulary*, the teacher and the children look together at the photocopied pictures, and the teacher names and talks about each illustration. The teacher then proceeds to read out the riddles as suggested above.

1   It has words in it. You can read it. (*book*)
2   It is hard. Dogs like to chew it. (*bone*)
3   It flies around your garden. It makes a buzzing noise. (*bee*)
4   You can play with this. You can kick it and bounce it. (*ball*)
5   Your coat might have some. They fit through holes. (*buttons*)
6   We have lips. A bird has this instead. (*beak*)
7   This is made of wood. You can hit a ball with it. (*bat*)
8   People ride on this. It has wheels. (*bus*)
9   You put things in this. It has a lid. (*box*)
10   This can fly. It has two legs. (*bird*)
11   It has sheets on it. It has a pillow on it. (*bed*)
12   You can fill it with water. You can wash in it. (*bath*)

Alliteration for the 'b' sound

Suitable for children in Years R, 1 and 2

→ The teacher states what the target sound is. They then read out each two-word phrase, and, after each one, the children must say whether one word or both words start with the target sound.

→ Alternatively, the teacher can give each child two cards with the target sound printed on. If both words in the phrase begin with the target sound, the children hold up two cards. If only one begins with that sound, they hold up one card.

beautiful butterfly	small button
big bone	bossy bird
bad cat	wooden bat
bald man	noisy bus
paper bag	busy bee
bold badger	square box

Tongue twisters for the 'b' sound

Suitable for children in Years R, 1 and 2

→ The teacher reads each tongue twister aloud and, after each one, asks the children to repeat it once or twice.

→ The children can play a game of Chinese Whispers. The teacher whispers the tongue twister to one child; this child whispers it to the next and so on. The last child says out loud what they think the teacher said, and this is compared with the original tongue twister.

1 Ben built a big blue boat.
2 Barry bought a big bunch of bananas for Bonita.
3 The beautiful butterfly balanced on the buttercup.
4 Bryony broke her brand new brown bracelet.
5 Blake, the blacksmith, blamed Black Beauty for his blister.

Odd word out — initial sounds

Involving words beginning with the 'b' sound

→ The children are told which initial sound to listen for. They then listen while the teacher reads aloud one line of three words at a time. After each line the children are asked to say which word did not begin with the target sound.

1	baby	cat	bear
2	bag	pig	bath
3	balloon	table	boat
4	boy	bell	doll
5	banana	bat	house
6	book	pen	basket
7	door	bottle	bee
8	bubble	bus	car
9	mouse	box	bird
10	bead	beach	coach
11	goat	bounce	belt
12	bull	bowl	pear
13	bicycle	biscuit	ring
14	summer	butter	button
15	bucket	cuckoo	butterfly

Odd word out – rhyming
Using a word beginning with the 'b' sound

→ The children are told to listen for the word that does not rhyme with the other two. They then listen while the teacher reads aloud one line of three words at a time. After each line the children are asked to say which word does not rhyme with the other two.

→ Alternatively, the children could be asked to say which two words do rhyme.

→ As an extra task, the children could think of other words that rhyme with the two rhyming words in each set.

1	hall	red	ball
2	coat	book	look
3	fair	bear	car
4	bed	hat	head
5	box	socks	feet
6	boat	bone	cone
7	sheet	bee	tea
8	well	bell	hall
9	bear	bead	stair
10	leg	bag	rag

Words to sound out for the 'b' sound

→ Only words with regular spelling have been included.

→ The teacher takes one word at a time and 'sounds out' each phoneme. This may need to be done several times. The children must then guess what the word is. Some children may be able to try writing the word.

→ The children may like to repeat the phonemes consecutively, just as the teacher did, to help them blend the sounds into words.

b—u—s	b—ea—k	b—ir—d	b—e—d
b—e—ll	b—oo—k	b—a—g	b—a—t

Story for the 'b' sound

→ The teacher asks the children to listen carefully to the story and pick out the words beginning with the target sound. The teacher then reads the story, sentence by sentence. After each sentence the teacher asks the children:
  - To say how many words they heard beginning with the given sound in that sentence.
  - To repeat the words they heard beginning with the target sound.
→ Alternatively, the teacher can slowly read the whole story, and the children can make a tally mark on a piece of paper every time they hear a word beginning with the target sound. The children can then count up how many words they have heard beginning with that sound and tell the teacher what those words are.

Bobby's birthday

It was Bobby's birthday. He wanted a bicycle for his birthday. Bobby was still asleep in bed. His baby brother cried and woke Bobby up. Bobby remembered that it was his birthday so he bounced out of bed. He opened some of the boxes placed at the foot of his bed. His friend Billy had given him a toy bulldozer. His sister Beth had given him a toy sailing boat, and his Aunty Bella had given him a book about badgers. But Bobby was disappointed because he could not see a bicycle. Then Bobby's mother told Bobby to go outside into the back garden. Bobby ran out of the back door into the back garden. There was a blue bicycle with balloons tied to the handlebars. On the balloons it said, 'Happy Birthday Bobby'.

Puzzle worksheet for the 'b' sound

Suitable for children in Years 1 and 2

Use the 'b' pictures to help you with these puzzles.

Unscramble the words below. They all begin with 'b'.

1 agb   **2** edb   **3** tbao   **4** ebra   **5** hbta

_____   _____   _____   _____   _____

Look for the 'b' words in the wordsearch below. They can read down or across. There are eight 'b' words of three letters or more.

c	b	e	c	w	b	h	t
b	a	k	j	b	e	d	v
g	l	z	x	k	a	p	o
f	l	b	a	q	k	u	d
b	o	a	t	l	w	y	b
r	u	g	u	b	o	n	e
p	h	d	f	j	c	m	a
b	a	n	a	n	a	h	r

Write down the words that you found:

1 _____   2 _____

3 _____   4 _____

5 _____   6 _____

7 _____   8 _____

13

Illustrations for the 'b' sound

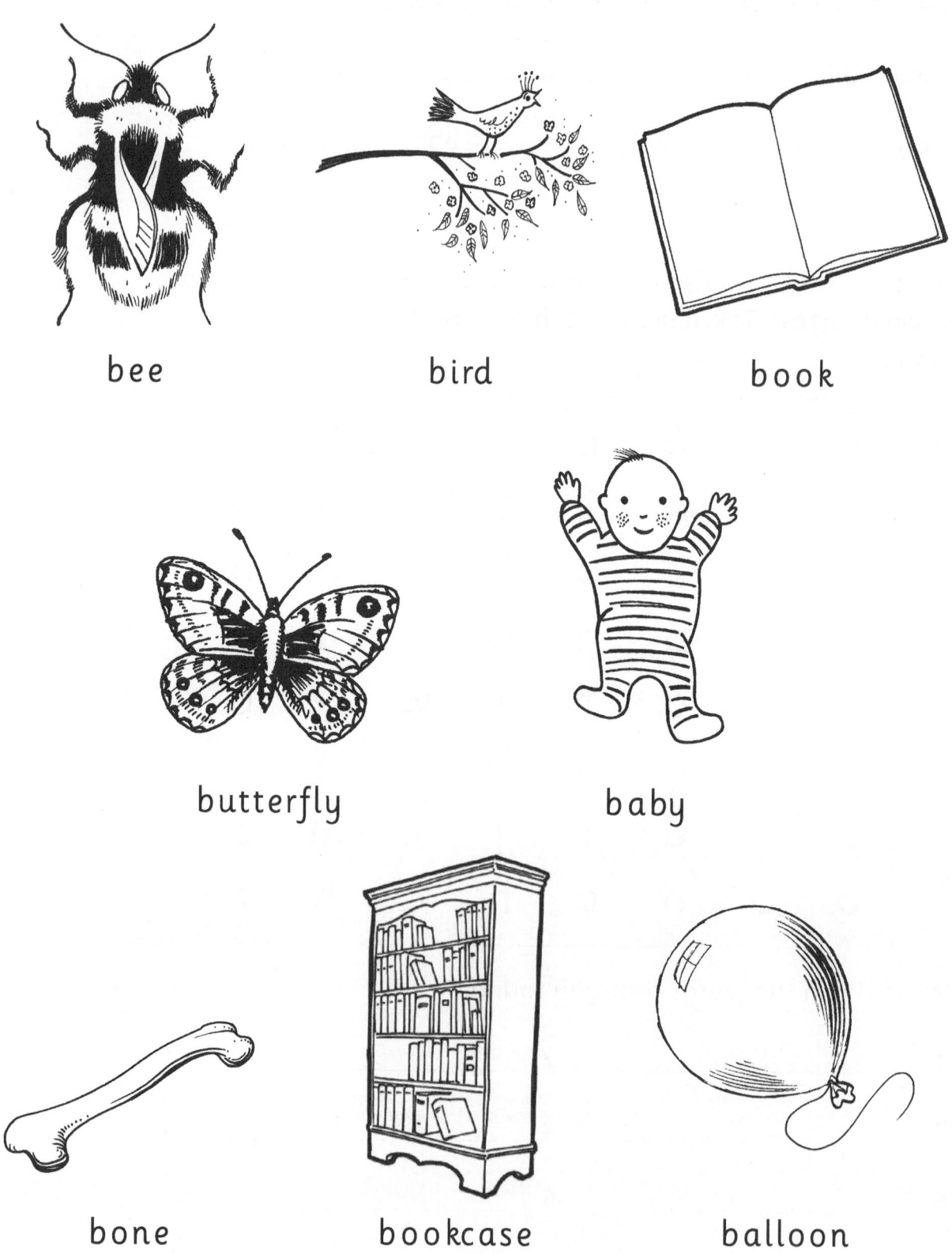

bee   bird   book

butterfly   baby

bone   bookcase   balloon

Illustrations for the 'b' sound

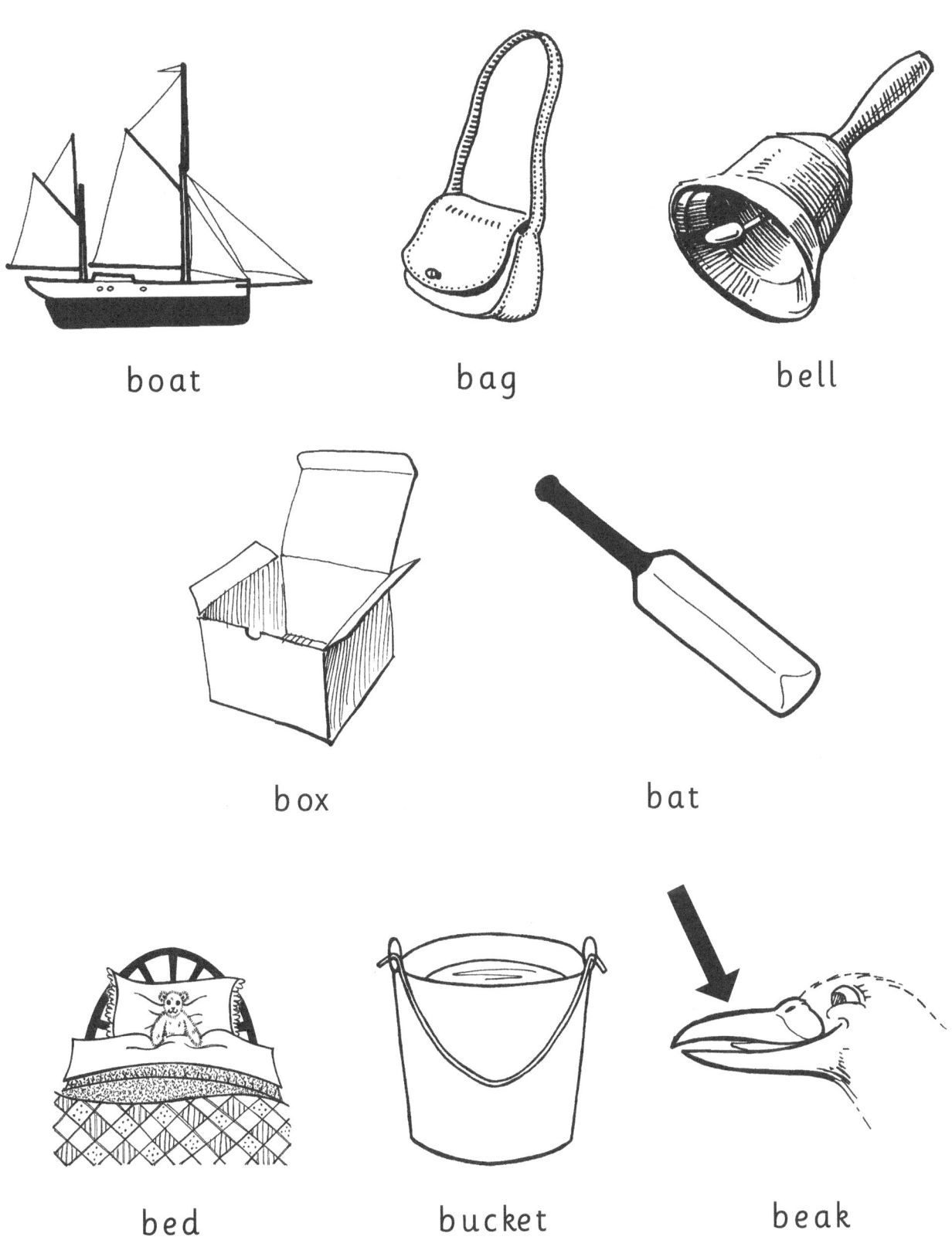

boat

bag

bell

box

bat

bed

bucket

beak

2/3

Illustrations for the 'b' sound

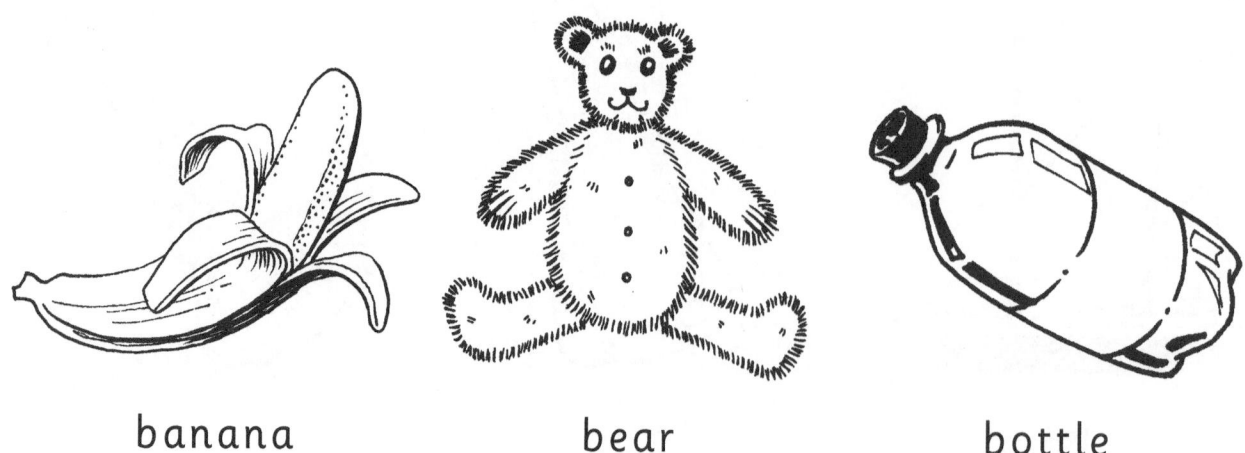

banana   bear   bottle

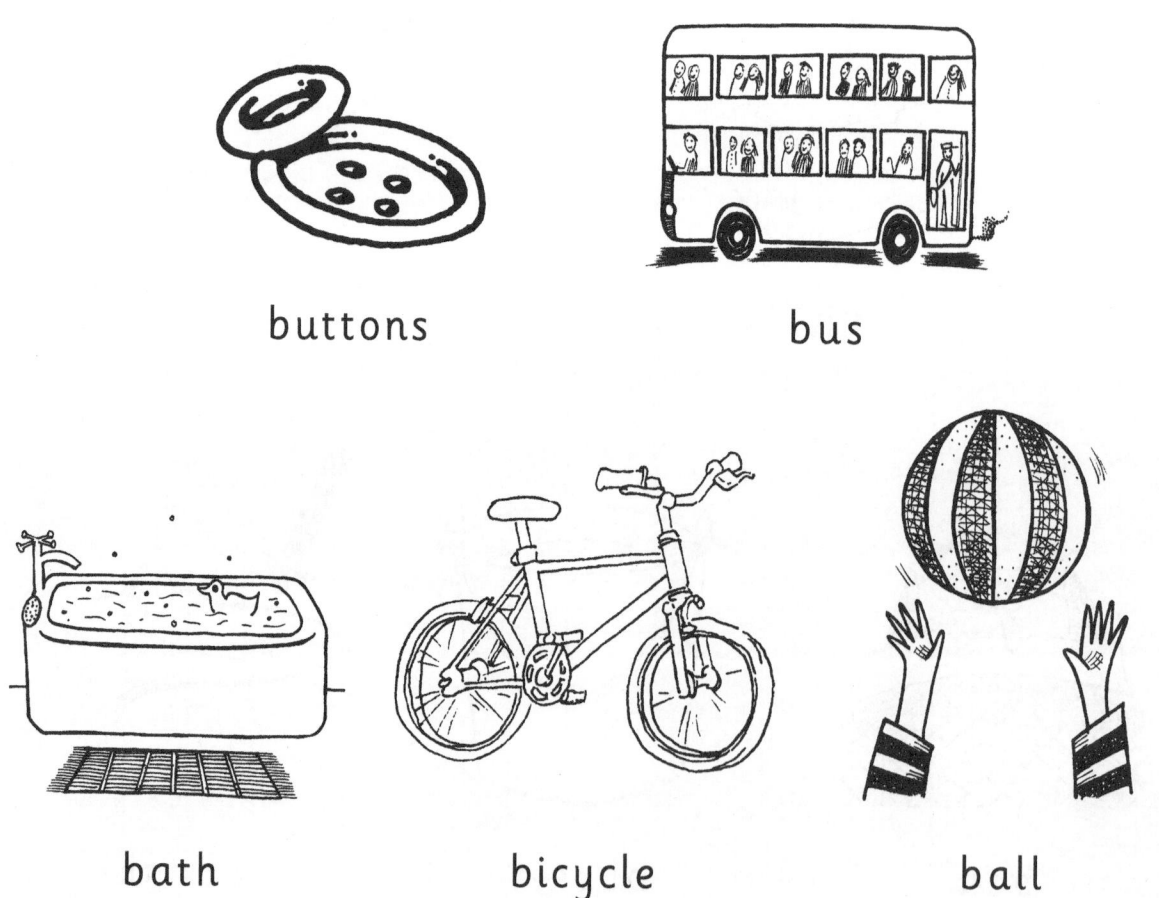

buttons   bus

bath   bicycle   ball

3/3

Section for the 'c/k' sound

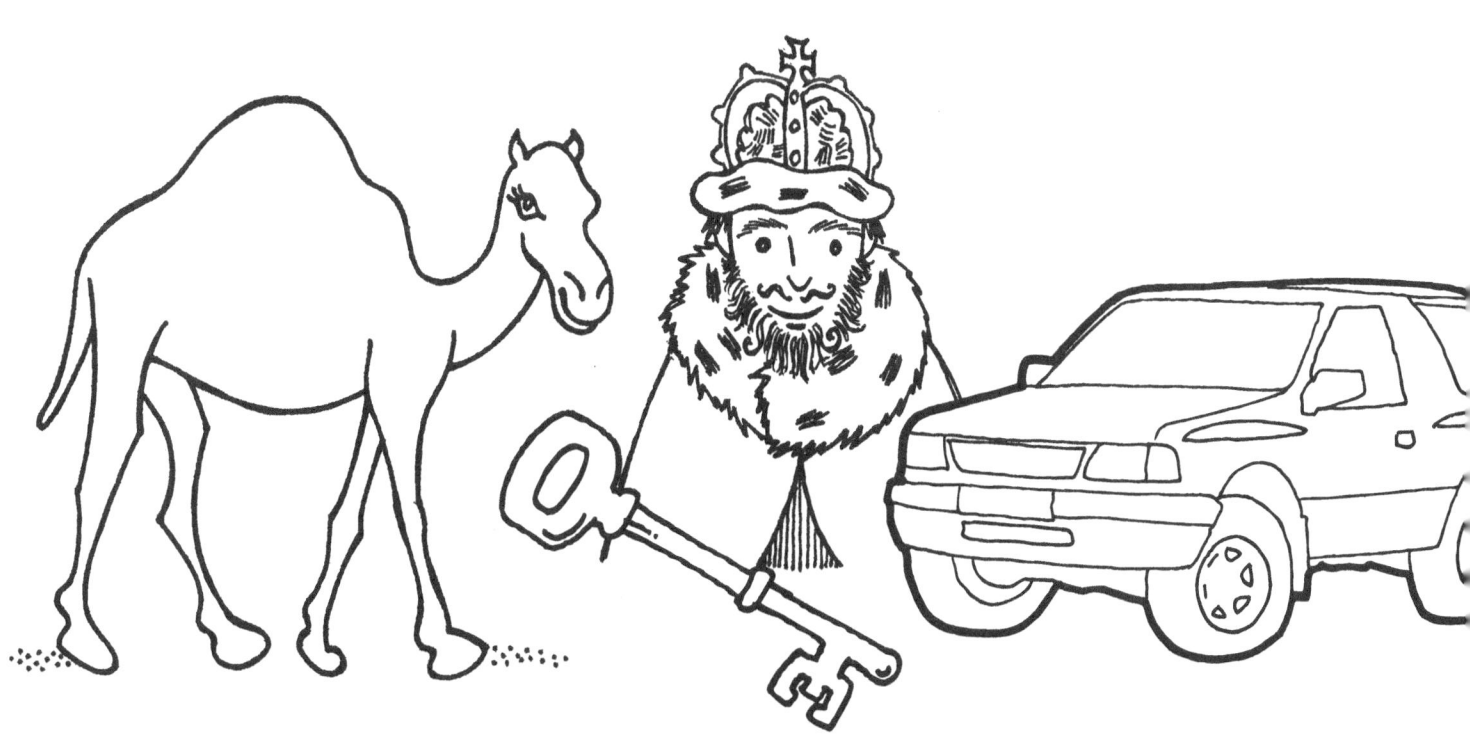

Section for the 'c/k' sound

Suitable for children in Year R

Riddles for the 'c/k' sound

→ Children are given the photocopied pictures to go with the target sound. The teacher reads out the riddles, one at a time, and the children decide which picture each one refers to. If desired, the children can then colour these pictures in.

→ *To make the activity more difficult*, the children, without access to the pictures, are told the target sound, and the riddles are read out one at a time. The children have to think of something that starts with that sound and fits in with the riddle.

→ *To teach vocabulary*, the teacher and the children look together at the photocopied pictures, and the teacher names and talks about each illustration. The teacher then proceeds to read out the riddles as suggested above.

1 This has a handle. You put it on a saucer. (*cup*)

2 You can eat this. It is an orange-coloured vegetable. (*carrot*)

3 It is made of wax. It has a flame. (*candle*)

4 This is an animal. It has a hump. (*camel*)

5 People stay in this for a holiday. It can move from place to place. (*caravan*)

6 This has teeth. It does not have a mouth. (*comb*)

7 You could put some ice-cream in one. You might see one on the road. (*cone*)

8 You thread this through a needle. You sew with it. (*cotton*)

9 You can eat it. It might have icing on it. (*cake*)

10 It is an animal. It might have horns. (*cow*)

11 This creature might wake us up. It makes a crowing noise. (*cockerel*)

12 It might have a collar or a hood. It keeps you warm in winter. (*coat*)

Alliteration for the 'c/k' sound

→ The teacher states what the target sound is. They then read out each two-word phrase, and, after each one, the children must say whether one word or both words start with the target sound.

→ Alternatively, the teacher can give each child two cards with the target sound printed on. If both words in the phrase begin with the target sound, the children hold up two cards. If only one begins with that sound, they hold up one card.

cold caravan	curly hair
colourful card	pink coat
corner cupboard	dark castle
cuddly camel	kicking kangaroo
kind girl	cookery book
careful carpenter	brown cow

Tongue twisters for the 'c/k' sound

→ The teacher reads each tongue twister aloud and, after each one, asks the children to repeat it once or twice.

→ The children can play a game of Chinese Whispers. The teacher whispers the tongue twister to one child; this child whispers it to the next and so on. The last child says out loud what they think the teacher said, and this is compared with the original tongue twister.

1 Carol cooked a carrot cake.
2 King Karl kept koalas and kangaroos.
3 Cody caught the cod and cooked it.
4 Custard, the cat, curled up on the curtains.
5 Claude and Clare climbed the clay cliff.

Odd word out — initial sounds

Involving words beginning with the 'c/k' sound

→ The children are told which initial sound to listen for. They then listen while the teacher reads aloud one line of three words at a time. After each line the children are asked to say which word did not begin with the target sound.

1	cup	dig	cow
2	cake	game	car
3	carrot	castle	table
4	camel	bus	cat
5	pen	coat	coffee
6	ship	cold	comb
7	cotton	sailor	collar
8	cut	cushion	gate
9	candle	saddle	cupboard
10	cobweb	cucumber	dinner
11	crack	salt	crash
12	wolf	clown	clock
13	crying	greedy	crayon
14	cloud	climb	mice
15	cockerel	tambourine	caravan

Odd word out – rhyming
Using a word beginning with the 'c/k' sound

→ The children are told to listen for the word that does not rhyme with the other two. They then listen while the teacher reads aloud one line of three words at a time. After each line the children are asked to say which word does not rhyme with the other two.

→ Alternatively, the children could be asked to say which two words do rhyme.

→ As an extra task, the children could think of other words that rhyme with the two rhyming words in each set.

1	cow	lock	now
2	cake	home	rake
3	cot	not	part
4	raw	claw	mug
5	horn	corn	sock
6	candle	metal	handle
7	cat	clock	sock
8	page	wave	cage
9	car	star	fur
10	card	heart	guard

Words to sound out for the 'c/k' sound

→ Only words with regular spelling have been included.

→ The teacher takes one word at a time and 'sounds out' each phoneme. This may need to be done several times. The children must then guess what the word is. Some children may be able to try writing the word.

→ The children may like to repeat the phonemes consecutively, just as the teacher did, to help them blend the sounds into words.

c—ar	c—u—p	c—a—t	c—ar—d
c—oa—t	c—o—t	c—or—n	c—l—o—ck

Story for the 'c/k' sound

→ The teacher asks the children to listen carefully to the story and pick out the words beginning with the target sound. The teacher then reads the story, sentence by sentence. After each sentence the teacher asks the children:

- To say how many words they heard beginning with the given sound in that sentence.
- To repeat the words they heard beginning with the target sound.

→ Alternatively, the teacher can slowly read the whole story, and the children can make a tally mark on a piece of paper every time they hear a word beginning with the target sound. The children can then count up how many words they have heard beginning with that sound and tell the teacher what those words are.

The village fête

Callum and Chloe went to a fête in a village near Cardiff. They jumped up and down on the bouncy castle and had a ride on a pony called Candy. Then Chloe had a go on the coconut shy. She threw coloured balls at the coconuts, but she could not hit any of them. Callum bought some candyfloss and got covered in a sticky mess. It was so cold that Callum and Chloe went home with their dad in the car. When they got home, they took off their coats and combed their hair. Mum had just cooked a cake, so they had a piece of cake and a cup of coffee. The cat climbed onto Callum's lap. Mum gave the baby a carrot to play with. The baby crawled over to Callum and stroked the cat with the carrot. The cat scratched the baby and made him cry. The cat jumped off Callum's lap, and his coffee spilt all over the carpet.

Puzzle worksheet for the 'c/k' sound

Use the 'c' pictures to help you with these puzzles.

Unscramble the words below. They all begin with 'c'.

1 tco   **2** atc   **3** ctoa   **4** aceg   **5** lccko

_____   _____   _____   _____   _____

Look for the 'c' words in the wordsearch below. They can read down or across. There are eight 'c' words of three letters or more.

c	m	b	n	z	l	j	g
a	f	s	c	o	a	t	p
m	i	c	o	t	y	r	w
e	q	e	b	r	u	o	a
l	c	o	w	x	f	h	c
k	z	v	e	b	n	g	a
c	o	m	b	s	j	v	g
t	f	t	p	c	a	k	e

Write down the words that you found:

1 _____   2 _____

3 _____   4 _____

5 _____   6 _____

7 _____   8 _____

23

Illustrations for the 'c/k' sound

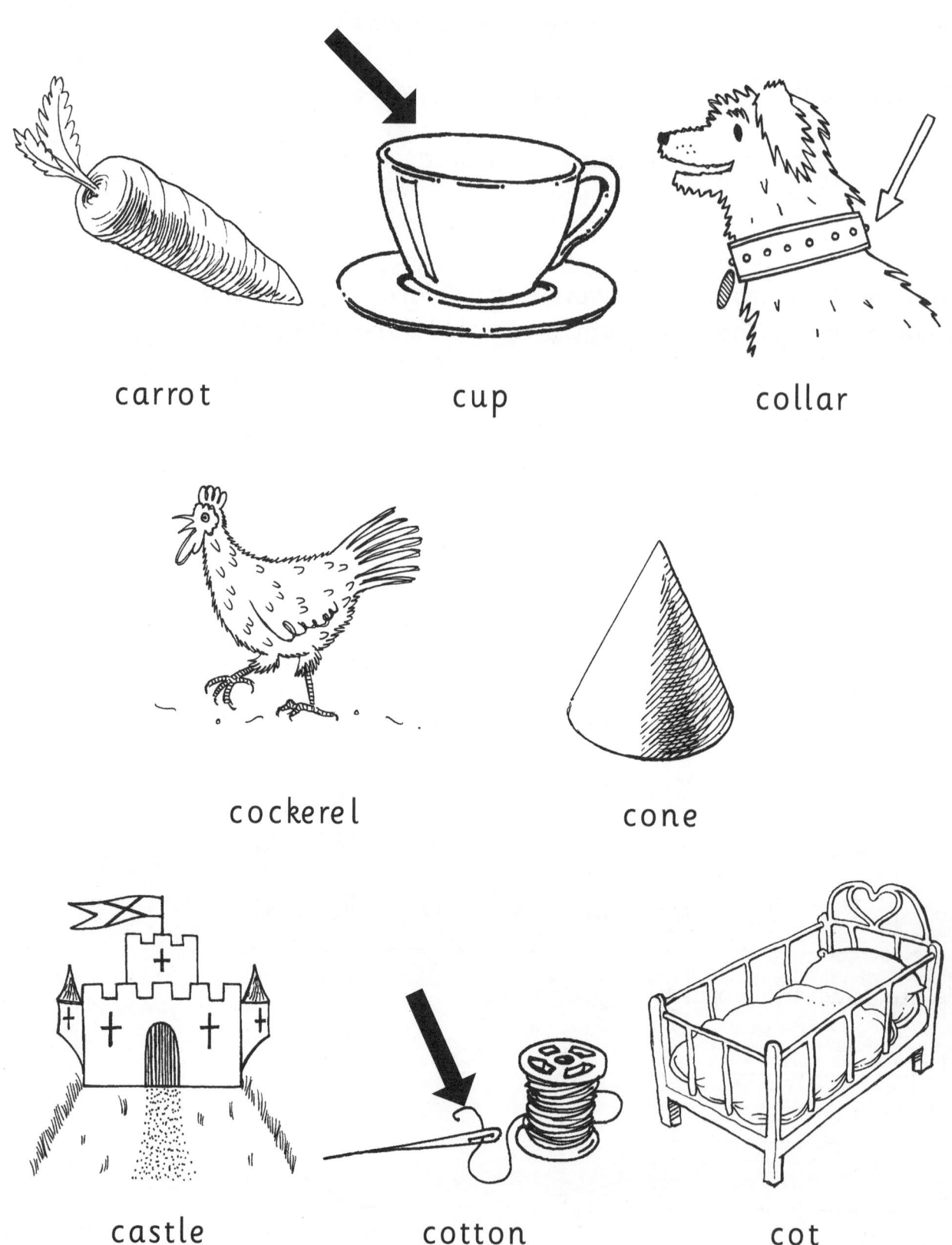

carrot

cup

collar

cockerel

cone

castle

cotton

cot

Illustrations for the 'c/k' sound

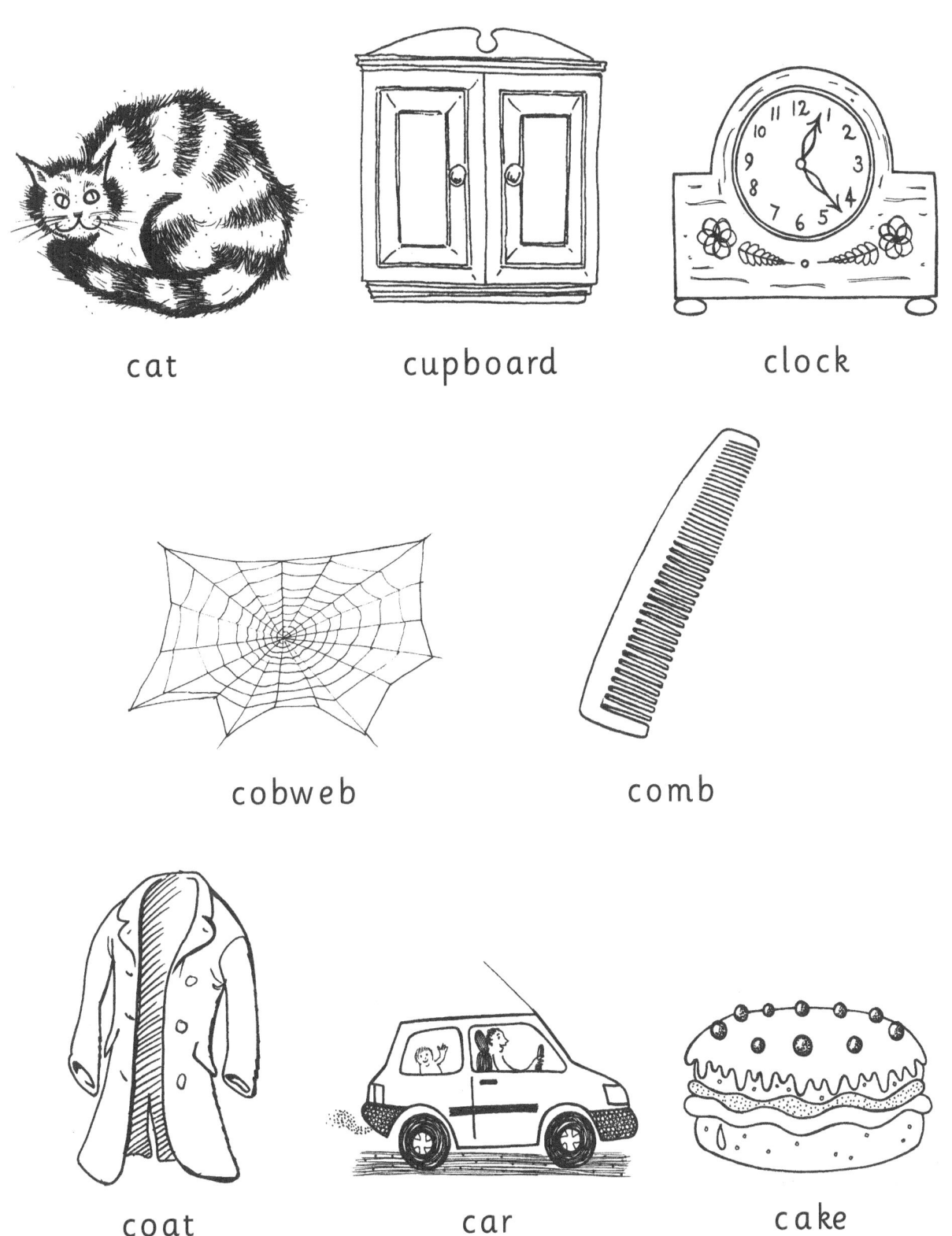

cat

cupboard

clock

cobweb

comb

coat

car

cake

2/3

Illustrations for the 'c/k' sound

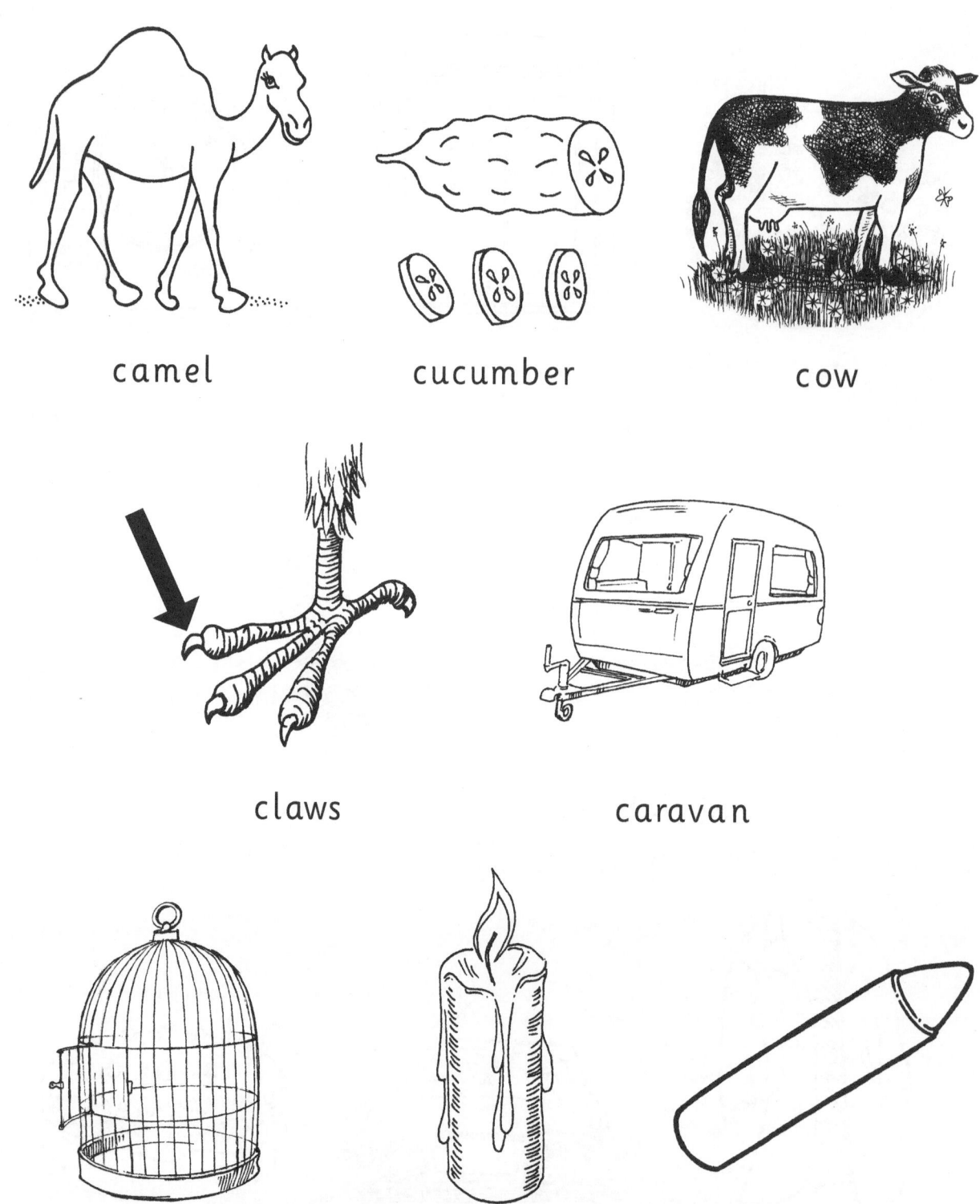

camel

cucumber

cow

claws

caravan

cage

candle

crayon

Section for the 'd' sound

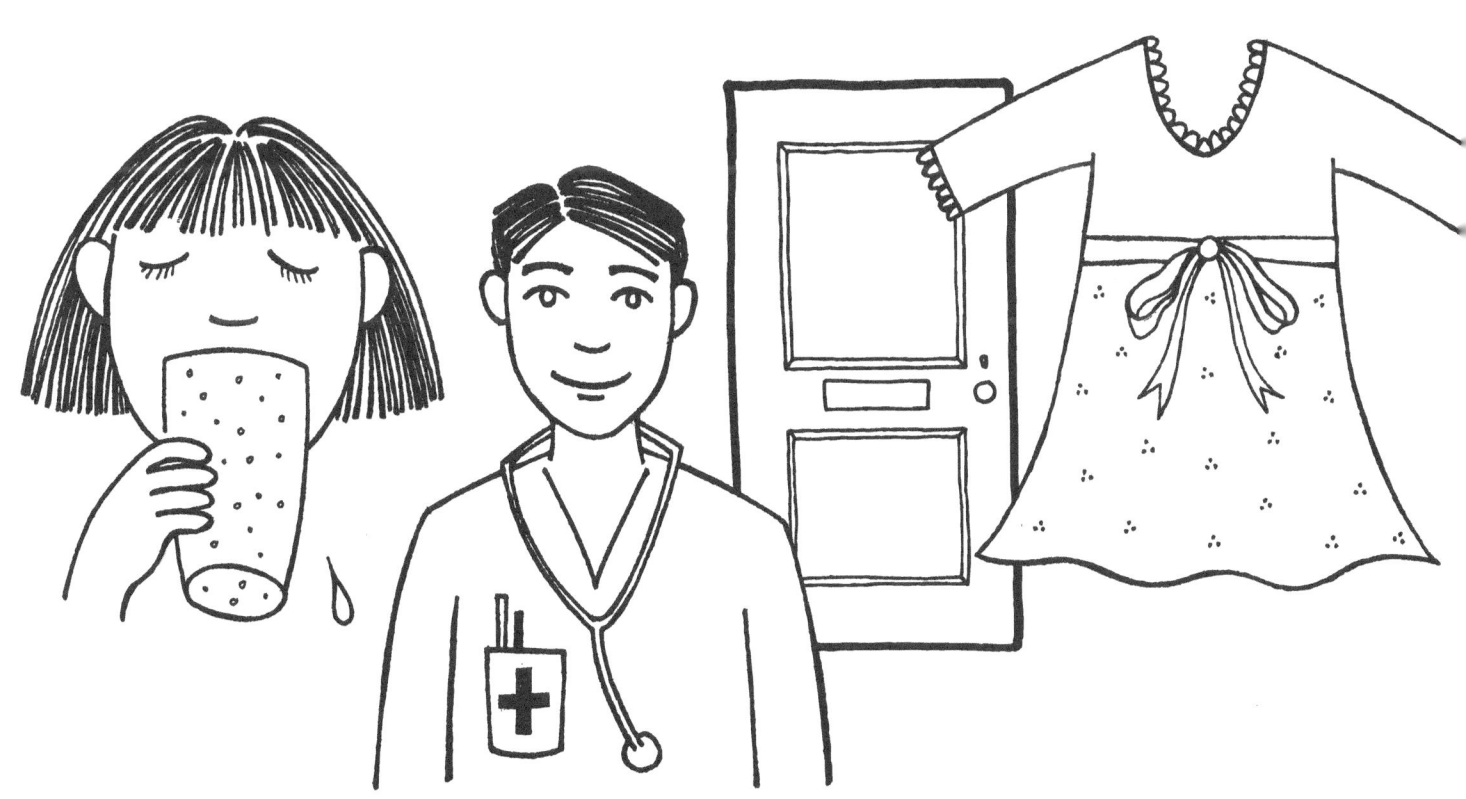

Section for the 'd' sound

Suitable for children in Year R

Riddles for the 'd' sound

→ Children are given the photocopied pictures to go with the target sound. The teacher reads out the riddles, one at a time, and the children decide which picture each one refers to. If desired, the children can then colour these pictures in.

→ *To make the activity more difficult*, the children, without access to the pictures, are told the target sound, and the riddles are read out one at a time. The children have to think of something that starts with that sound and fits in with the riddle.

→ *To teach vocabulary*, the teacher and the children look together at the photocopied pictures, and the teacher names and talks about each illustration. The teacher then proceeds to read out the riddles as suggested above.

1 This is an animal. It lived a long time ago. (*dinosaur*)
2 You might play with this. It might wear a dress. (*doll*)
3 You throw these in a game. They have numbers on them. (*dice*)
4 You might find this in a field. It has white petals. (*daisy*)
5 This is an animal. It has horns called antlers. (*deer*)
6 This is a person. You go to see them when you are ill. (*doctor*)
7 This can be made of wood. It has a handle. (*door*)
8 This has two legs and a beak. It likes swimming. (*duck*)
9 This is an animal. It usually lives in a field. (*donkey*)
10 You throw this in a game. It is very sharp. (*dart*)
11 This is a man or a woman. They look after your teeth. (*dentist*)
12 You can eat out of it. You might put cereal in it. (*dish*)

Alliteration for the 'd' sound

→ The teacher states what the target sound is. They then read out each two-word phrase, and, after each one, the children must say whether one word or both words start with the target sound.

→ Alternatively, the teacher can give each child two cards with the target sound printed on. If both words in the phrase begin with the target sound, the children hold up two cards. If only one begins with that sound, they hold up one card.

dirty donkey	deep river
fizzy drink	dusty dice
wooden door	dark cave
fierce dog	dangerous dinosaur
purple dish	dead deer
different dessert	sharp dart

Tongue twisters for the 'd' sound

→ The teacher reads each tongue twister aloud and, after each one, asks the children to repeat it once or twice.

→ The children can play a game of Chinese Whispers. The teacher whispers the tongue twister to one child; this child whispers it to the next and so on. The last child says out loud what they think the teacher said, and this is compared with the original tongue twister.

1 Dainty Deena dusted a dozen dirty doorsteps.
2 Declan decided to dig up the daisies.
3 Drake dropped his drumstick down the drain.
4 The drowsy driver drove over the drawbridge.
5 The drummer dreamed about a dreadful dragon.

Odd word out — initial sounds

Involving words beginning with the 'd' sound

→ The children are told which initial sound to listen for. They then listen while the teacher reads aloud one line of three words at a time. After each line the children are asked to say which word did not begin with the target sound.

1	duck	bun	dark
2	doll	torch	dug
3	cake	dance	dog
4	dice	down	gate
5	daisy	nose	deep
6	jaw	dish	deer
7	desk	chop	dot
8	dull	door	light
9	dart	toad	dig
10	girl	dot	desk
11	drum	rub	dress
12	doctor	taller	duster
13	dinner	dentist	kennel
14	jumper	digger	donkey
15	danger	garden	daddy

30

Odd word out – rhyming
Using a word beginning with the 'd' sound

→ The children are told to listen for the word that does not rhyme with the other two. They then listen while the teacher reads aloud one line of three words at a time. After each line the children are asked to say which word does not rhyme with the other two.

→ Alternatively, the children could be asked to say which two words do rhyme.

→ As an extra task, the children could think of other words that rhyme with the two rhyming words in each set.

1	dart	heart	cot
2	down	foal	brown
3	kite	dice	mice
4	tall	drill	fill
5	less	dress	nest
6	door	tar	four
7	fair	deer	near
8	wish	dish	rash
9	daisy	juicy	lazy
10	bank	drink	sink

Words to sound out for the 'd' sound

→ Only words with regular spelling have been included.

→ The teacher takes one word at a time and 'sounds out' each phoneme. This may need to be done several times. The children must then guess what the word is. Some children may be able to try writing the word.

→ The children may like to repeat the phonemes consecutively, just as the teacher did, to help them blend the sounds into words.

d—o—g	d—i—sh	d—o—t	d—u—ck
d—o—ll	d—ar—t	d—ow—n	d—e—s—k

Story for the 'd' sound

→ The teacher asks the children to listen carefully to the story and pick out the words beginning with the target sound. The teacher then reads the story, sentence by sentence. After each sentence the teacher asks the children:
  - To say how many words they heard beginning with the given sound in that sentence.
  - To repeat the words they heard beginning with the target sound.
→ Alternatively, the teacher can slowly read the whole story, and the children can make a tally mark on a piece of paper every time they hear a word beginning with the target sound. The children can then count up how many words they have heard beginning with that sound and tell the teacher what those words are.

Dilly the donkey

Daniel and Dinah lived on a farm. Daniel kept a pet donkey called Dilly, and Dinah had a pet duck called Duke. They were also fond of Dougal, the dog, who looked after the dopey sheep. One day, Dilly the donkey was not in his field when Daniel went to give him his dinner. Daniel saw that the fence had been damaged and that there was a hole in it big enough for Dilly to get through. Daniel was worried because the donkey might be in danger. Then Dinah shouted to Daniel that Duke, the duck, was not in his pond. They looked everywhere for Dilly and Duke. Suddenly Daniel noticed the donkey and the duck. The duck was sitting on the donkey's back. The donkey was standing in a dirty ditch eating the daises and daffodils from the bank. The doctor was visiting their dad, who was ill. Daniel asked the doctor to help them to drag the donkey out of the ditch.

Puzzle worksheet for the 'd' sound

Suitable for children in Years 1 and 2

Use the 'd' pictures to help you with these puzzles.

Unscramble the words below. They all begin with 'd'.

1 gdo   **2** dllo   **3** cdei   **4** cdku   **5** edre

_____   _____   _____   _____   _____

Look for the 'd' words in the wordsearch below. They can read down or across. There are eight 'd' words of three letters or more.

z	c	b	m	d	v	x	d
d	l	j	d	o	l	l	i
i	d	h	f	n	s	a	n
n	a	v	g	k	h	p	o
n	i	d	r	e	s	s	s
e	s	u	t	y	e	r	a
r	y	q	d	u	c	k	u
s	j	g	k	d	o	o	r

Write down the words that you found:

1 _____   2 _____

3 _____   4 _____

5 _____   6 _____

7 _____   8 _____

33

Illustrations for the 'd' sound

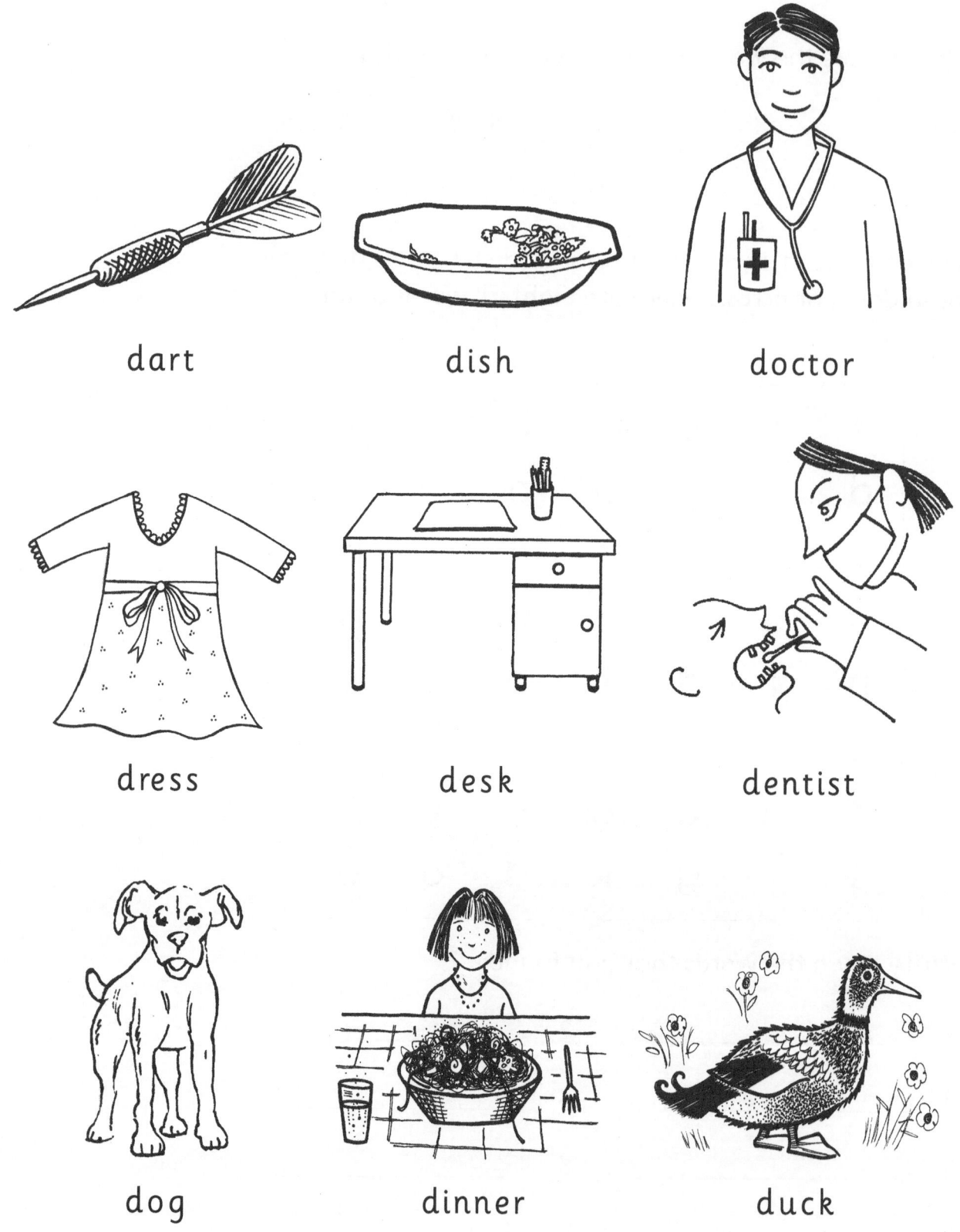

dart

dish

doctor

dress

desk

dentist

dog

dinner

duck

Illustrations for the 'd' sound

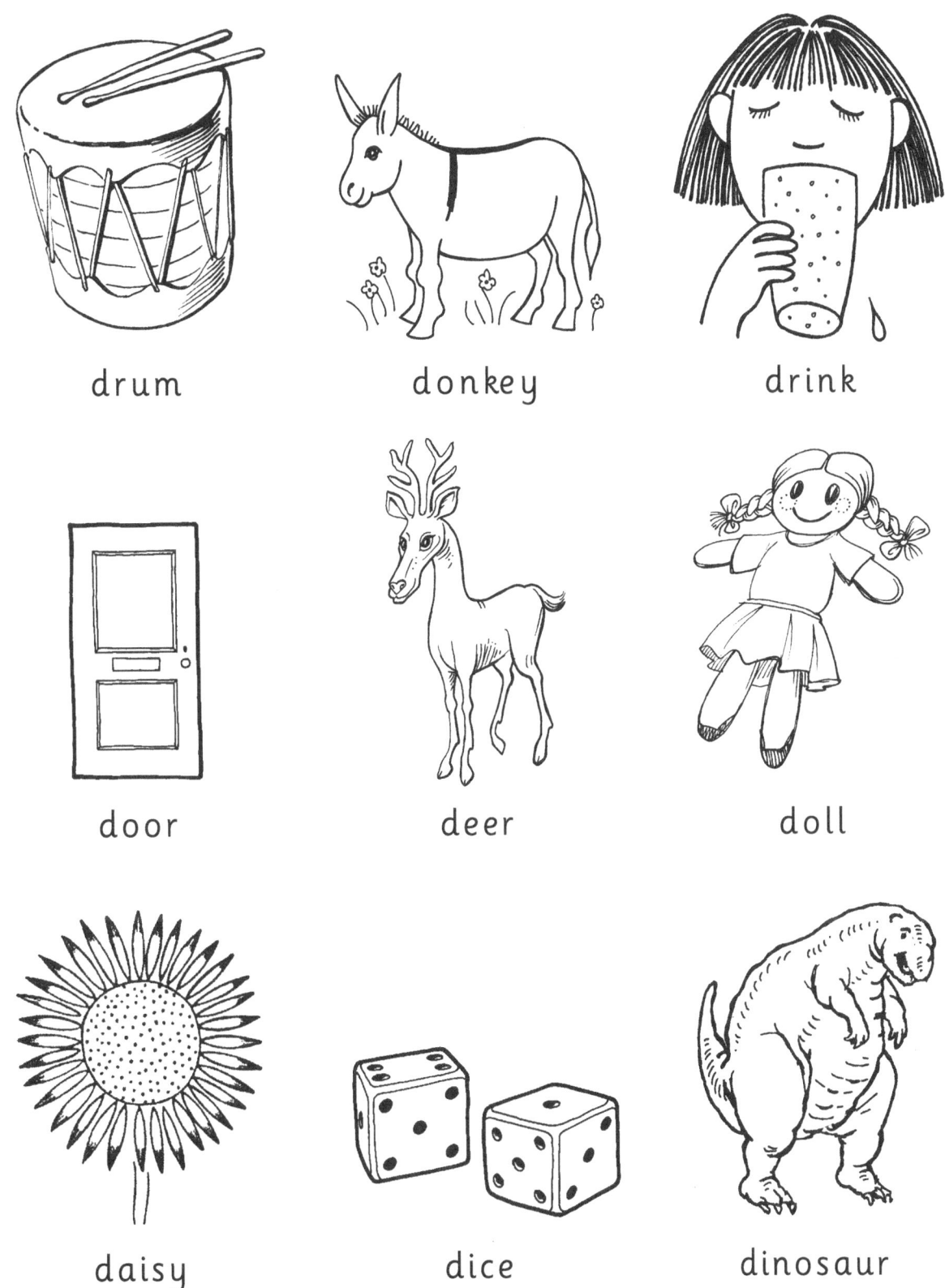

drum

donkey

drink

door

deer

doll

daisy

dice

dinosaur

2/2

Section for the 'f' sound

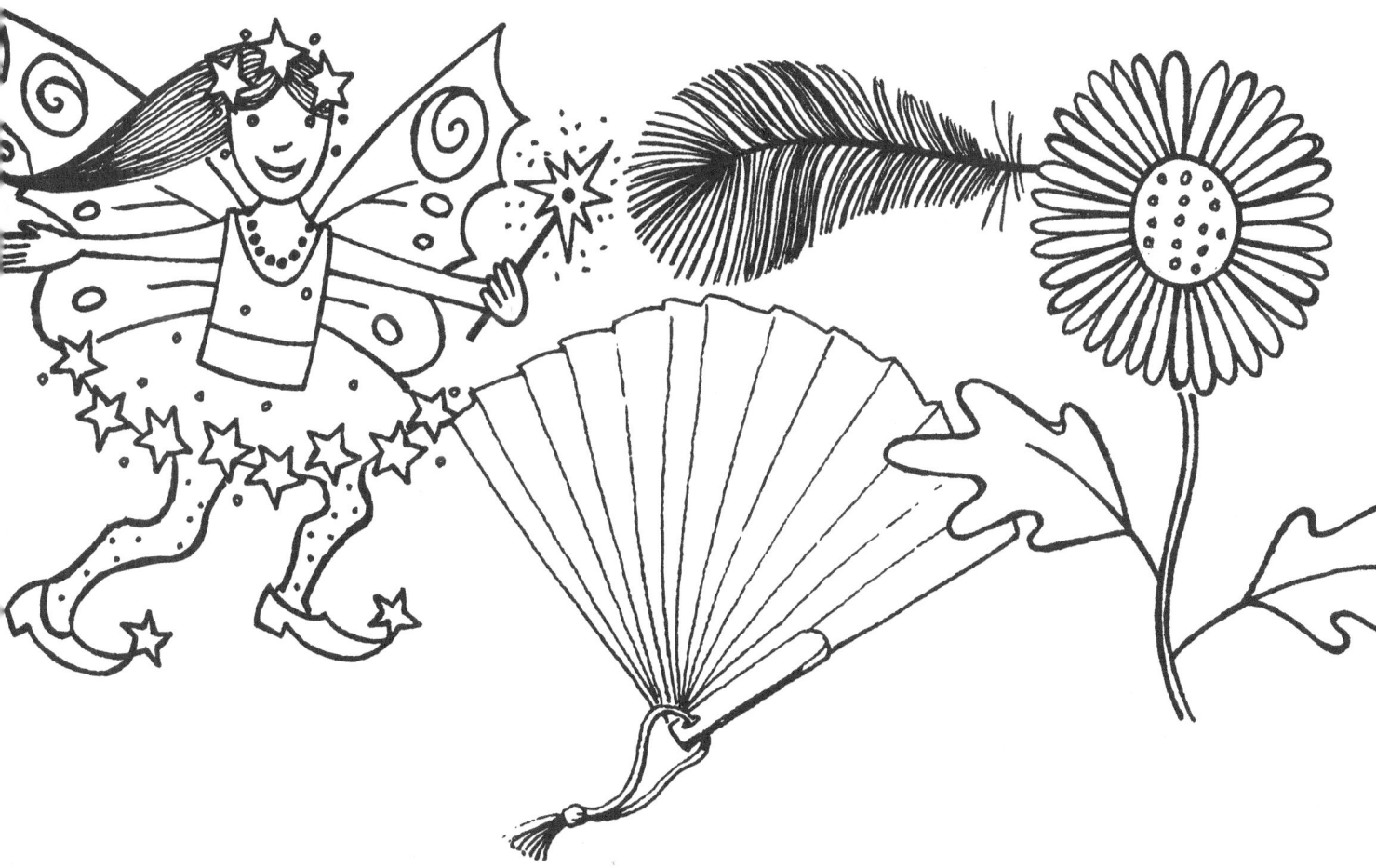

Section for the 'f' sound

Riddles for the 'f' sound

→ Children are given the photocopied pictures to go with the target sound. The teacher reads out the riddles, one at a time, and the children decide which picture each one refers to. If desired, the children can then colour these pictures in.

→ *To make the activity more difficult*, the children, without access to the pictures, are told the target sound, and the riddles are read out one at a time. The children have to think of something that starts with that sound and fits in with the riddle.

→ *To teach vocabulary*, the teacher and the children look together at the photocopied pictures, and the teacher names and talks about each illustration. The teacher then proceeds to read out the riddles as suggested above.

1   This is a number. A dog has this many legs. (*four*)
2   It has prongs. It has a handle. (*fork*)
3   You have five toes on this. It is at the end of your leg. (*foot*)
4   This is an animal. He went after the Little Red Hen. (*fox*)
5   You might throw this. You might kick it. (*football*)
6   This has eyes and a mouth. It has fins as well. (*fish*)
7   This is a number. You have as many toes as this on each foot. (*five*)
8   This is an animal. You could ride it when it is grown up. (*foal*)
9   This has eyes and a nose. It also has cheeks and a chin. (*face*)
10 It might go around your garden. It might have a gate in it. (*fence*)
11 It is like a doll. It holds a magic wand. (*fairy*)
12 You hold this in your hand. You wave it to keep yourself cool. (*fan*)

Alliteration for the 'f' sound

→ The teacher states what the target sound is. They then read out each two-word phrase, and, after each one, the children must say whether one word or both words start with the target sound.

→ Alternatively, the teacher can give each child two cards with the target sound printed on. If both words in the phrase begin with the target sound, the children hold up two cards. If only one begins with that sound, they hold up one card.

filthy football	funny clown
four fish	fizzy water
fast car	long finger
fierce fox	fat foal
wooden fence	five sheep
forty fireworks	fresh fruit

Tongue twisters for the 'f' sound

→ The teacher reads each tongue twister aloud and, after each one, asks the children to repeat it once or twice.

→ The children can play a game of Chinese Whispers. The teacher whispers the tongue twister to one child; this child whispers it to the next and so on. The last child says out loud what they think the teacher said, and this is compared with the original tongue twister.

1 Fay fetched her four favourite fantastic fireworks.
2 Felicity found the fat foal in the farmer's furthest field.
3 Florence flopped onto the fabulous flat floor.
4 The fly flew from the floating flower to the flagpole.
5 Franklyn fried some frozen fish fingers.

Odd word out — initial sounds

Involving words beginning with the 'f' sound

→ The children are told which initial sound to listen for. They then listen while the teacher reads aloud one line of three words at a time. After each line the children are asked to say which word did not begin with the target sound.

1	four	pet	fan
2	shop	fish	five
3	thumb	face	food
4	fork	fall	bull
5	fence	light	fire
6	vase	foal	fox
7	fun	pan	fin
8	met	fat	full
9	found	played	foot
10	sleep	flag	fleece
11	frog	rag	freeze
12	finger	feather	window
13	fairy	battle	football
14	flannel	antler	flower
15	fourteen	fifteen	sixteen

Odd word out – rhyming
Using a word beginning with the 'f' sound

Suitable for children in Years R, 1 and 2

→ The children are told to listen for the word that does not rhyme with the other two. They then listen while the teacher reads aloud one line of three words at a time. After each line the children are asked to say which word does not rhyme with the other two.

→ Alternatively, the children could be asked to say which two words do rhyme.

→ As an extra task, the children could think of other words that rhyme with the two rhyming words in each set.

1	fan	ham	can
2	star	four	more
3	fork	pork	dark
4	fat	vet	pat
5	foot	soot	cool
6	fire	hare	tyre
7	pig	frog	dog
8	five	dive	cave
9	lace	mice	face
10	foal	coal	tail

Words to sound out for the 'f' sound

Suitable for children in Years R, 1 and 2

→ Only words with regular spelling have been included.

→ The teacher takes one word at a time and 'sounds out' each phoneme. This may need to be done several times. The children must then guess what the word is. Some children may be able to try writing the word.

→ The children may like to repeat the phonemes consecutively, just as the teacher did, to help them blend the sounds into words.

f—a—n	f—i—sh	f—i—n	f—or—k
f—oo—t	f—oa—l	f—oo—d	f—ee—t

Story for the 'f' sound

→ The teacher asks the children to listen carefully to the story and pick out the words beginning with the target sound. The teacher then reads the story, sentence by sentence. After each sentence the teacher asks the children:
  – To say how many words they heard beginning with the given sound in that sentence.
  – To repeat the words they heard beginning with the target sound.
→ Alternatively, the teacher can slowly read the whole story, and the children can make a tally mark on a piece of paper every time they hear a word beginning with the target sound. The children can then count up how many words they have heard beginning with that sound and tell the teacher what those words are.

The foggy night

It was a freezing, foggy night. Filip and Finlay were walking home. They were fourteen-year-old twins and they lived on a farm. Filip and Finlay were taking a short cut across the fields to their farm. There was a full moon, which was hidden by the freezing fog. They tried to find the path across Mr Ferry's wheat field. When they could not find the path, they tried to feel for the fence. If they could find the fence, they could follow it around to the gate. But Filip and Finlay could not see or feel anything. Their father had told them to be home by 10 o'clock. Filip and Finlay knew that their father would be worried about them. They were both frightened as they were lost in the freezing fog. Then Filip saw a fuzzy shape in the fog. It looked like a fox. Finlay said that it could be the same fox that had stolen one of their father's chickens on Friday night. Filip and Finlay guessed that the fox was going back to the farmyard to try and steal another chicken. They managed to follow the fox, and they reached their farm safely. However, when Filip, Finlay and their father went back outside to find the fox, it had fled.

Puzzle worksheet for the 'f' sound

Use the 'f' pictures to help you with these puzzles.

Unscramble the words below. They all begin with 'f'.

1 anf   **2** ylf   **3** ofru   **4** frok   **5** sifh

_____   _____   _____   _____   _____

Look for the 'f' words in the wordsearch below. They can read down or across. There are eight 'f' words of three letters or more.

a	s	f	d	f	z	x	f
c	q	o	w	f	e	r	a
f	g	u	h	e	f	i	n
o	j	r	k	a	m	b	g
r	l	m	v	t	c	f	e
k	f	i	s	h	x	l	r
z	w	p	g	e	s	y	v
f	a	c	e	r	x	j	w

Write down the words that you found:

1 _____   2 _____

3 _____   4 _____

5 _____   6 _____

7 _____   8 _____

43

Illustrations for the 'f' sound

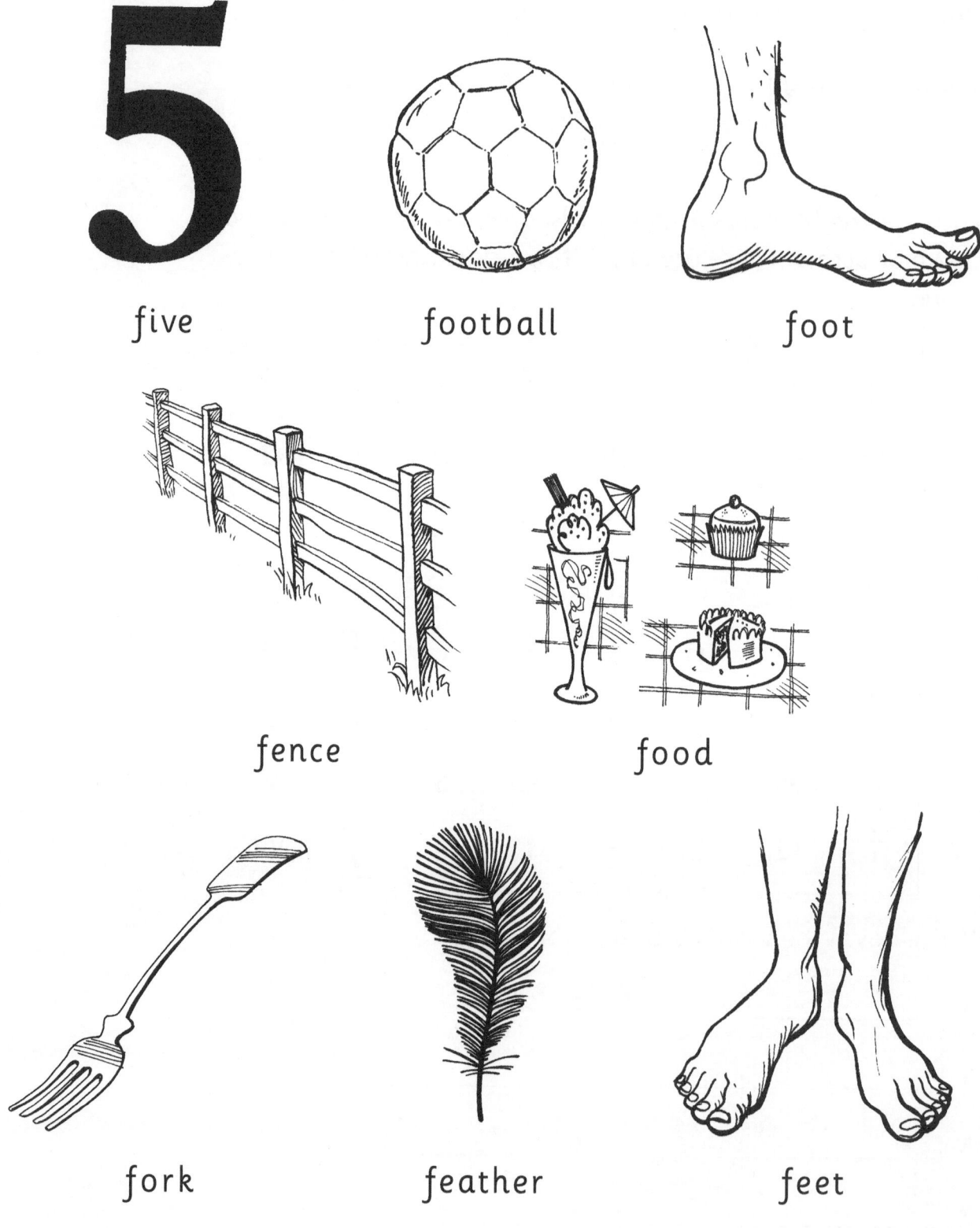

five

football

foot

fence

food

fork

feather

feet

Illustrations for the 'f' sound

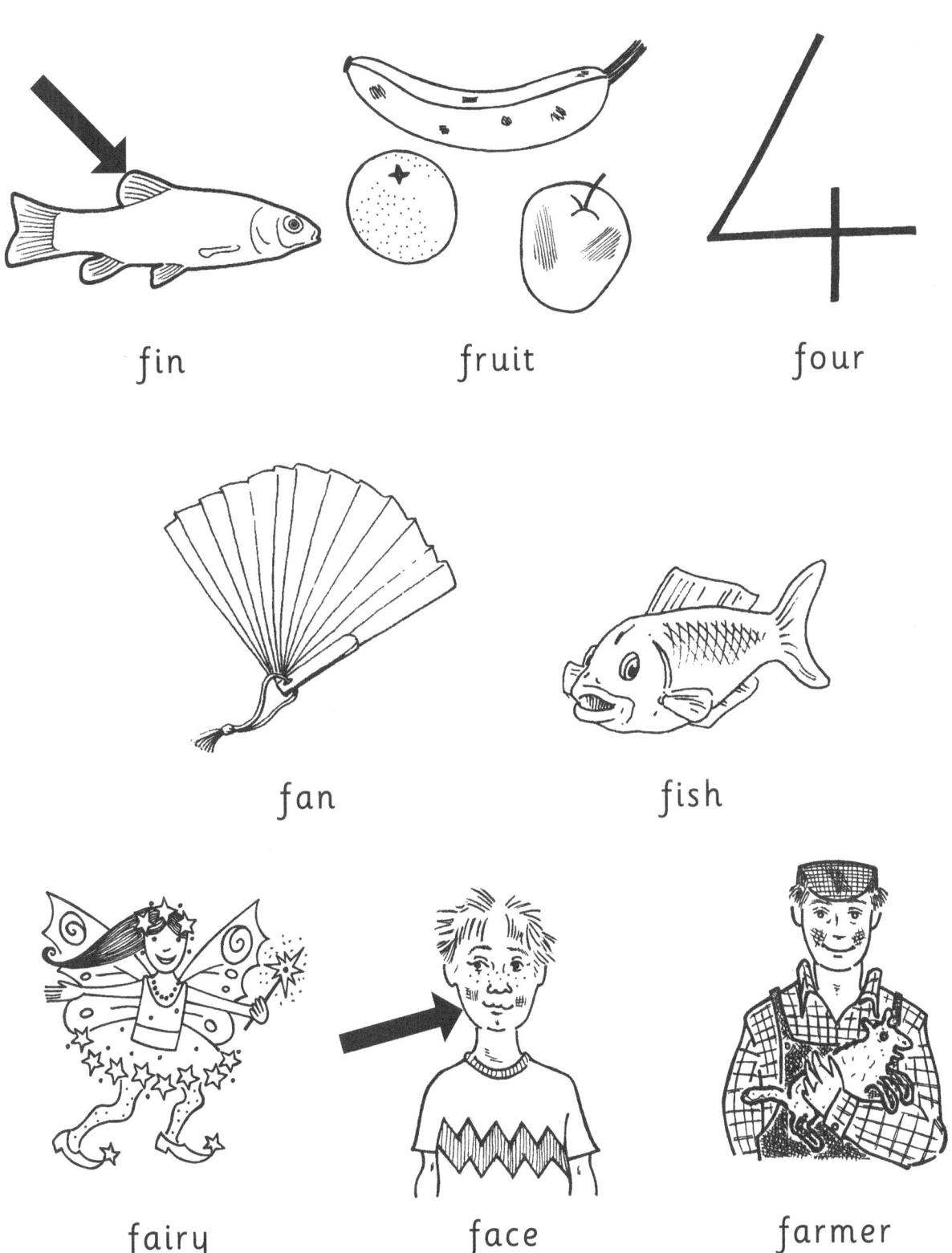

fin   fruit   four

fan   fish

fairy   face   farmer

2/3

Illustrations for the 'f' sound

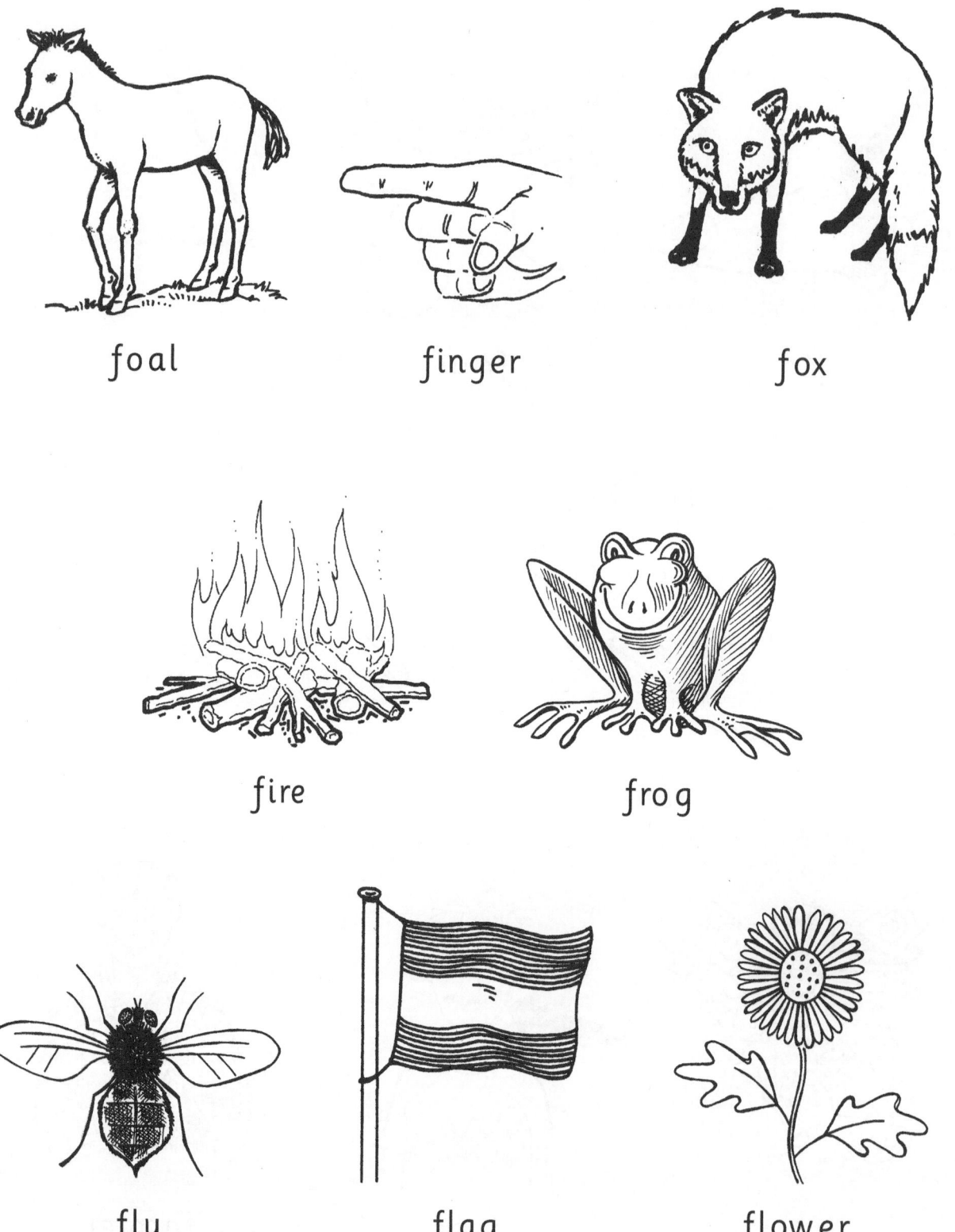

foal   finger   fox

fire   frog

fly   flag   flower

Section for the 'g' sound

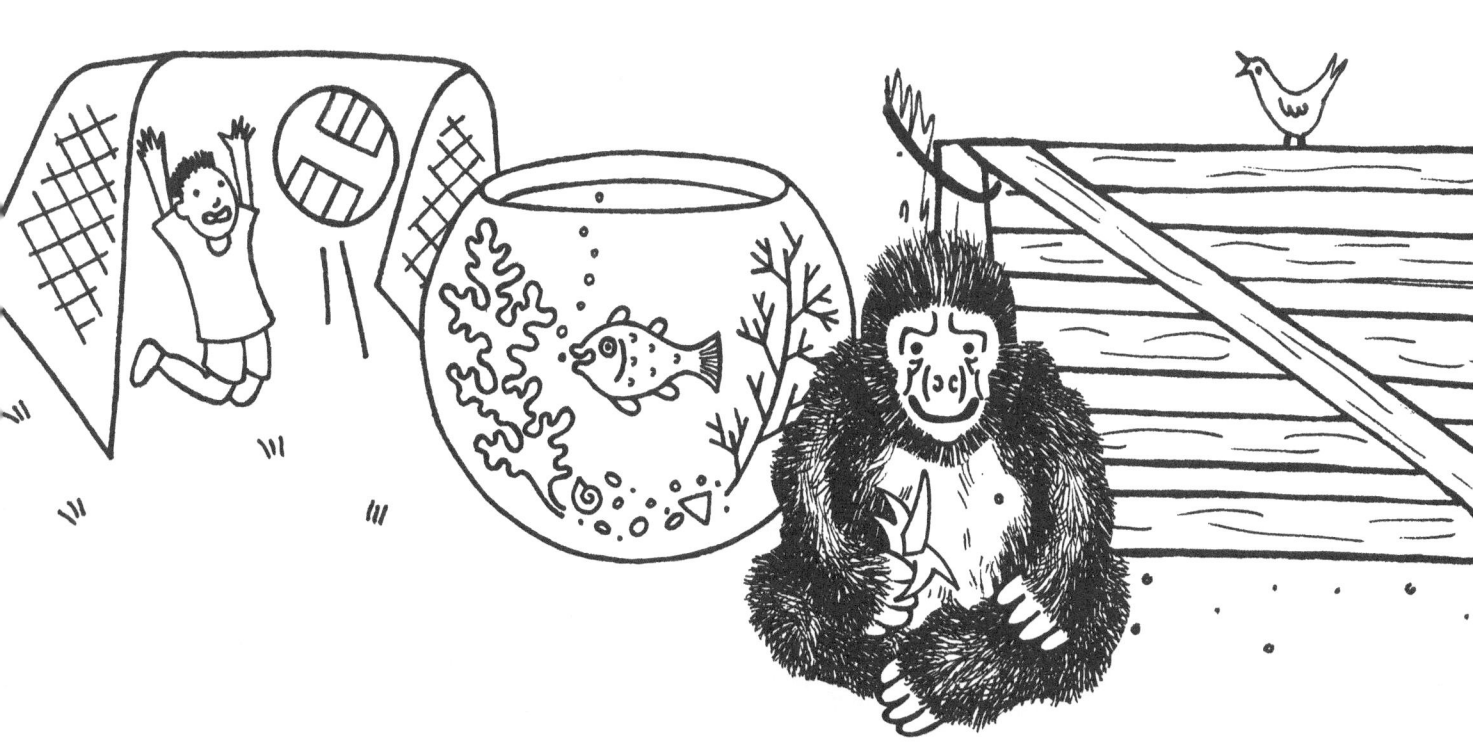

Section for the 'g' sound

Riddles for the 'g' sound

→ Children are given the photocopied pictures to go with the target sound. The teacher reads out the riddles, one at a time, and the children decide which pictures each one refers to. If desired, the children can then colour these pictures in.

→ *To make the activity more difficult*, the children, without access to the pictures, are told the target sound, and the riddles are read out one at a time. The children have to think of something that starts with that sound and fits in with the riddle.

→ *To teach vocabulary*, the teacher and the children look together at the photocopied pictures, and the teacher names and talks about each illustration. The teacher then proceeds to read out the riddles as suggested above.

1 It is orange in colour. It might live in a tank or a bowl. (*goldfish*)
2 It might have flowers and grass in it. It might have a path. (*garden*)
3 It has posts and a net. You kick a ball into it. (*goal*)
4 It is a building. Cars are kept in it. (*garage*)
5 This lays eggs. It looks like a duck. (*goose*)
6 You can play this. It has strings. (*guitar*)
7 It is usually white. You might dress up as one for Halloween. (*ghost*)
8 This animal has a beard. It might also have horns. (*goat*)
9 This might have a latch. You open and shut it. (*gate*)
10 You can play this. It might have counters and dice. (*game*)
11 It is green. You cut it when it grows too long. (*grass*)
12 These are fruit. They grow in bunches. (*grapes*)

Alliteration for the 'g' sound

➜ The teacher states what the target sound is. They then read out each two-word phrase, and, after each one, the children must say whether one word or both words start with the target sound.

➜ Alternatively, the teacher can give each child two cards with the target sound printed on. If both words in the phrase begin with the target sound, the children hold up two cards. If only one begins with that sound, they hold up one card.

good goat	gorgeous flowers
silly goose	friendly ghost
garden gate	ghastly gorilla
gold guitar	brick garage
girl guide	funny goggles
glittering glasses	green grapes

Tongue twisters for the 'g' sound

➜ The teacher reads each tongue twister aloud and, after each one, asks the children to repeat it once or twice.

➜ The children can play a game of Chinese Whispers. The teacher whispers the tongue twister to one child; this child whispers it to the next and so on. The last child says out loud what they think the teacher said, and this is compared with the original tongue twister.

1 Gail gave some garlic to Guy, the gorilla.
2 Gilbert, the goat, galloped around the garden.
3 Gloria glued her gloves to her glamorous glasses.
4 Greta grew grapes in the greenhouse for her granny.
5 Greg's grandad grumbled and groaned.

Odd word out – initial sounds

Involving words beginning with the 'g' sound

→ The children are told which initial sound to listen for. They then listen while the teacher reads aloud one line of three words at a time. After each line the children are asked to say which word did not begin with the target sound.

1	goal	fan	gate
2	time	go	gift
3	gum	gas	call
4	road	goose	goat
5	girl	world	get
6	guard	nine	golf
7	game	ghost	heart
8	sat	give	got
9	grape	meat	green
10	cots	gloves	glass
11	group	grey	dice
12	tripped	grumbled	groaned
13	garage	carpet	garden
14	guitar	goldfish	dolphin
15	tulip	garlic	gallop

Odd word out – rhyming
Using a word beginning with the 'g' sound

→ The children are told to listen for the word that does not rhyme with the other two. They then listen while the teacher reads aloud one line of three words at a time. After each line the children are asked to say which word does not rhyme with the other two.

→ Alternatively, the children could be asked to say which two words do rhyme.

→ As an extra task, the children could think of other words that rhyme with the two rhyming words in each set.

1	gate	jump	date
2	dress	ghost	toast
3	girl	first	pearl
4	cloud	goat	coat
5	green	tree	bean
6	plate	great	hat
7	plug	gown	town
8	game	stool	lame
9	rude	glue	blue
10	glove	grass	love

Words to sound out for the 'g' sound

→ Only words with regular spelling have been included.

→ The teacher takes one word at a time and 'sounds out' each phoneme. This may need to be done several times. The children must then guess what the word is. Some children may be able to try writing the word.

→ The children may like to repeat the phonemes consecutively, just as the teacher did, to help them blend the sounds into words.

g—oa—t	g—ir—l	g—i—f—t	g—oa—l
g—r—ee—n	g—r—i—n	g—l—a—d	g—r—a—n

Story for the 'g' sound

→ The teacher asks the children to listen carefully to the story and pick out the words beginning with the target sound. The teacher then reads the story, sentence by sentence. After each sentence the teacher asks the children:
  – To say how many words they heard beginning with the given sound in that sentence.
  – To repeat the words they heard beginning with the target sound.
→ Alternatively, the teacher can slowly read the whole story, and the children can make a tally mark on a piece of paper every time they hear a word beginning with the target sound. The children can then count up how many words they have heard beginning with that sound and tell the teacher what those words are.

Halloween night

Grace and Gabbie Gilpin were going to a Halloween ghost party at Guy's house. The girls put on white gowns and white gloves. They painted their faces with green face paint that glowed in the dark. Their granny called to see them, and they gave her quite a fright. It was getting dark, and it was time for the ghost party. The girls decided to take the path through the graveyard to Guy's house. Grace and Gabbie opened the gate to the gloomy graveyard and closed it behind them. The girls met a group of boys walking along the stony ground. The boys were grinning and laughing. Their grins disappeared as they gazed at two ghastly ghosts. Suddenly the boys gave a great cry. They galloped over the gravestones and dived through a gap in the hedge. Grace and Gabbie grinned at each other. The day before, one of the group of boys had deliberately thrown grey paint over Grace's new green glasses.

Puzzle worksheet for the 'g' sound

Use the 'g' pictures to help you with these puzzles.

Unscramble the words below. They all begin with 'g'.

1 otag   **2** tgea   **3** grli   **4** gsoeo   **5** olveg

_____   _____   _____   _____   _____

Look for the 'g' words in the wordsearch below. They can read down or across. There are eight 'g' words of three letters or more.

g	a	m	e	m	b	g	c
o	l	u	j	g	o	a	t
a	g	g	p	h	i	r	y
l	r	u	n	o	w	d	q
z	s	i	d	s	x	e	v
g	a	t	e	t	g	n	f
d	a	a	p	l	m	x	w
h	g	r	a	p	e	s	v

Write down the words that you found:

1 _____   2 _____

3 _____   4 _____

5 _____   6 _____

7 _____   8 _____

53

Illustrations for the 'g' sound

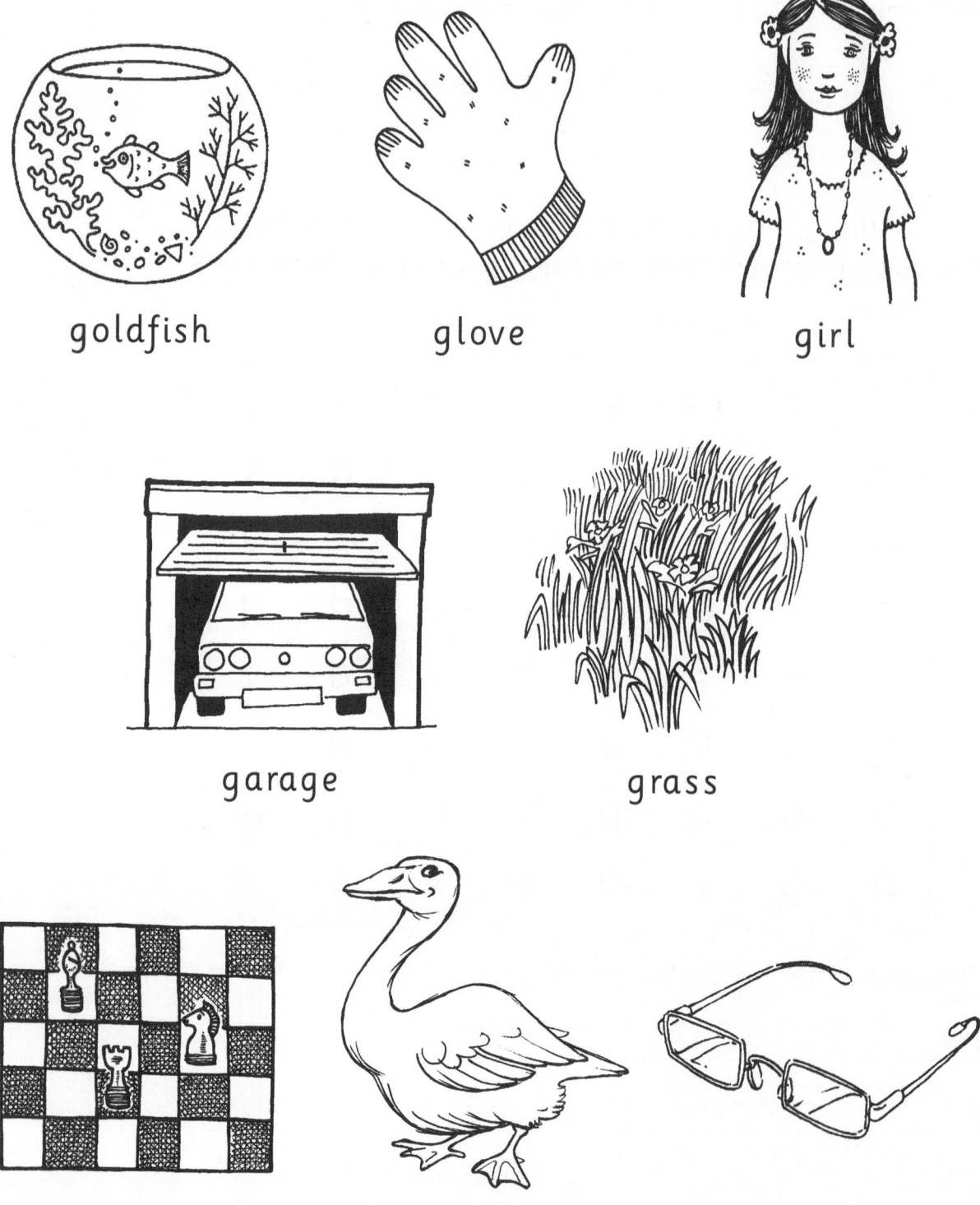

goldfish

glove

girl

garage

grass

game

goose

glasses

Illustrations for the 'g' sound

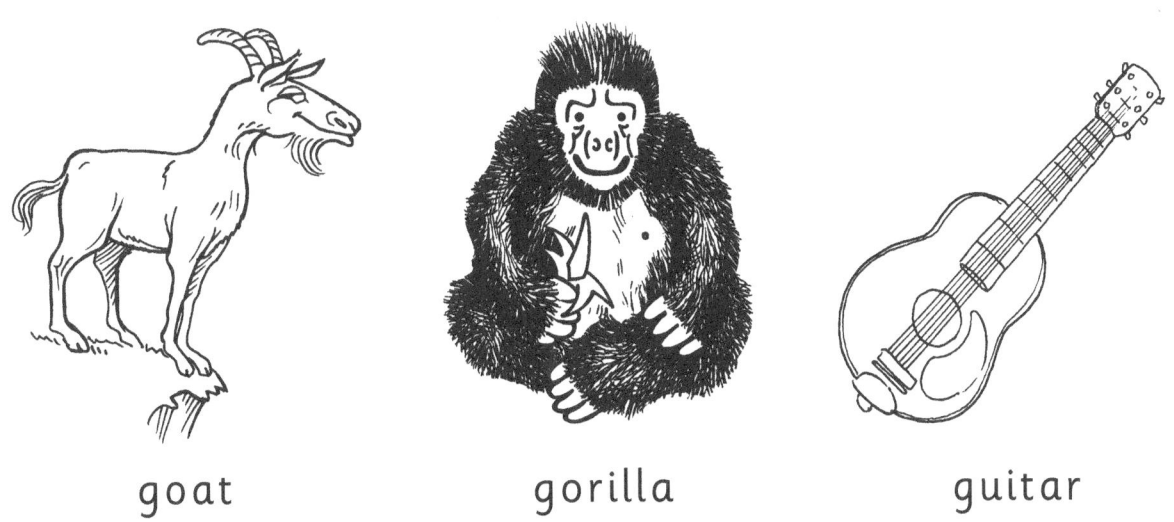

goat   gorilla   guitar

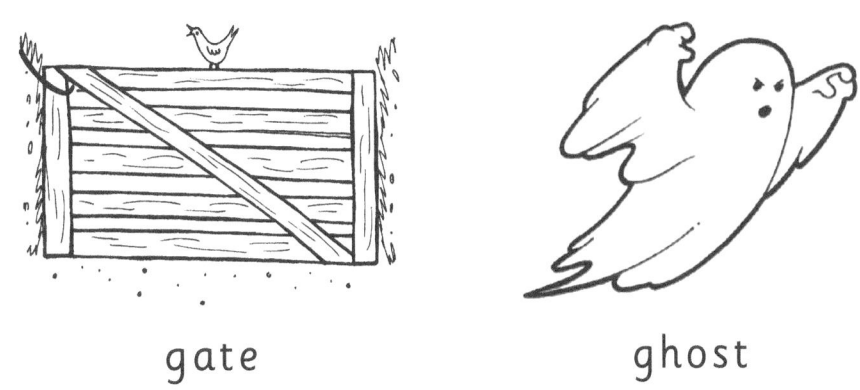

gate   ghost

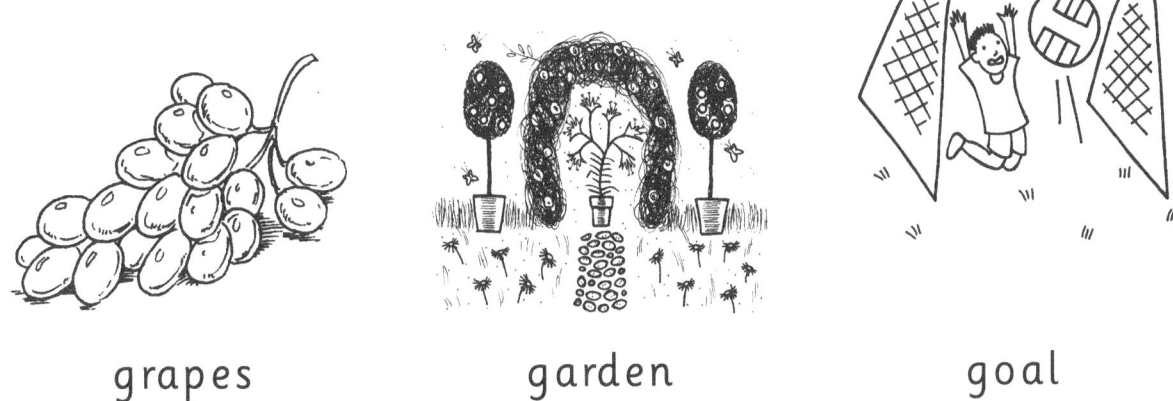

grapes   garden   goal

2/2

Routledge Taylor & Francis Group

Section for the 'h' sound

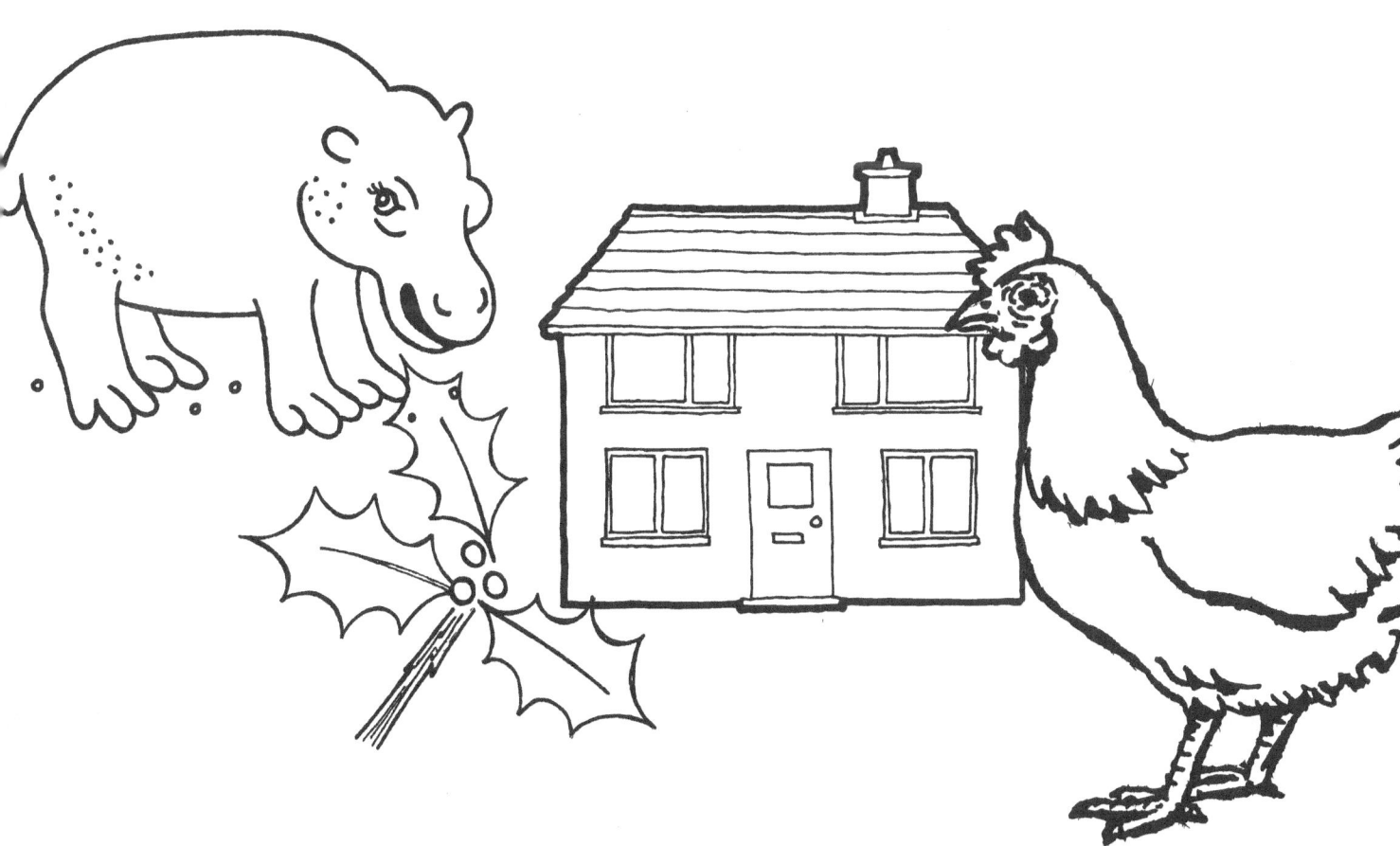

Section for the 'h' sound

Suitable for children in Year R

Riddles for the 'h' sound

→ Children are given the photocopied pictures to go with the target sound. The teacher reads out the riddles, one at a time, and the children decide which picture each one refers to. If desired, the children can then colour these pictures in.

→ *To make the activity more difficult*, the children, without access to the pictures, are told the target sound, and the riddles are read out one at a time. The children have to think of something that starts with that sound and fits in with the riddle.

→ *To teach vocabulary*, the teacher and the children look together at the photocopied pictures, and the teacher names and talks about each illustration. The teacher then proceeds to read out the riddles as suggested above.

1 You walk on this. It is part of your foot. (*heel*)
2 This is a building. You see doctors and nurses here. (*hospital*)
3 You might hang your coat on it. You might catch fish with it. (*hook*)
4 This is an animal. It has a mane and a tail. (*horse*)
5 You can walk up this. You can walk down this. (*hill*)
6 This is part of your body. It is just below your waist. (*hip*)
7 This has a hook. You put clothes on it. (*hanger*)
8 This cannot swim or fly in the sky. It lays eggs for us to eat. (*hen*)
9 This is part of your body. It is joined to your neck. (*head*)
10 A lady might carry one. She keeps money and other things in it. (*handbag*)
11 This is part of your body. It is joined to your wrist. (*hand*)
12 This is a large animal. It lives in water and on land. (*hippo*)

Alliteration for the 'h' sound

→ The teacher states what the target sound is. They then read out each two-word phrase, and, after each one, the children must say whether one word or both words start with the target sound.

→ Alternatively, the teacher can give each child two cards with the target sound printed on. If both words in the phrase begin with the target sound, the children hold up two cards. If only one begins with that sound, they hold up one card.

happy hippo	long hair
horrible horse	heavy hammer
huge house	hard biscuit
red heart	hot toast
high hill	spiky hedgehog
hungry hamster	sticky honey

Tongue twisters for the 'h' sound

→ The teacher reads each tongue twister aloud and, after each one, asks the children to repeat it once or twice.

→ The children can play a game of Chinese Whispers. The teacher whispers the tongue twister to one child; this child whispers it to the next and so on. The last child says out loud what they think the teacher said, and this is compared with the original tongue twister.

1 Hazel's hat hung on the hook in the hall.
2 Hagrid, the happy horse, hurt his hoof on the holly.
3 Hannah and Harry hid in the highest hammock.
4 Hunter had a horrible hairy hound.
5 Honey had a hungry hamster in her handbag.

Odd word out – initial sounds

Involving words beginning with the 'h' sound

→ The children are told which initial sound to listen for. They then listen while the teacher reads aloud one line of three words at a time. After each line the children are asked to say which word did not begin with the target sound.

1	hand	fair	hen
2	hat	head	girl
3	chair	hop	house
4	horse	hit	pond
5	hill	wolf	hole
6	toy	hook	half
7	heel	hide	thin
8	hair	deer	hang
9	hard	hurt	art
10	hold	ill	high
11	pear	hear	help
12	hammer	turkey	heavy
13	rabbit	hungry	hanger
14	hippo	helmet	kitchen
15	helicopter	telephone	hospital

Odd word out — rhyming
Using a word beginning with the 'h' sound

→ The children are told to listen for the word that does not rhyme with the other two. They then listen while the teacher reads aloud one line of three words at a time. After each line the children are asked to say which word does not rhyme with the other two.

→ Alternatively, the children could be asked to say which two words do rhyme.

→ As an extra task, the children could think of other words that rhyme with the two rhyming words in each set.

1	hair	spade	fair
2	van	heel	feel
3	hook	look	door
4	hill	fill	well
5	land	hen	pen
6	hat	bat	cot
7	hand	send	band
8	map	hip	lip
9	head	dad	bed
10	house	sauce	mouse

Words to sound out for the 'h' sound

→ Only words with regular spelling have been included.

→ The teacher takes one word at a time and 'sounds out' each phoneme. This may need to be done several times. The children must then guess what the word is. Some children may be able to try writing the word.

→ The children may like to repeat the phonemes consecutively, just as the teacher did, to help them blend the sounds into words.

h—a—t	h—oo—k	h—ee—l	h—i—p
h—e—n	h—i—ll	h—a—n—d	h—a—m

Story for the 'h' sound

→ The teacher asks the children to listen carefully to the story and pick out the words beginning with the target sound. The teacher then reads the story, sentence by sentence. After each sentence the teacher asks the children:

 – To say how many words they heard beginning with the given sound in that sentence.

 – To repeat the words they heard beginning with the target sound.

→ Alternatively, the teacher can slowly read the whole story, and the children can make a tally mark on a piece of paper every time they hear a word beginning with the target sound. The children can then count up how many words they have heard beginning with that sound and tell the teacher what those words are.

Hamish the hamster

Heidi was happy to be going on holiday with her friend Heather and Heather's parents. They left Heather's house at 8 o'clock in the morning and got to the hotel at 3 o'clock that afternoon. Heidi and Heather helped to carry the heavy suitcases to their hotel room. The handle of Heidi's case came off and the case fell open. Out of the case hopped Hamish, Heidi's hamster. Heidi did not know how the hamster had got into the suitcase. Heidi and Heather hurried around the room after Hamish and managed to catch him. They found a picnic hamper belonging to Heather's mother. They put the hamster into Heather's mother's hamper. They made holes in the lid of the hamper so Hamish could breathe. Heidi hid the hamper under some hangers in the huge wardrobe. The hamster lived happily in this hamper during their stay at the hotel. Every time Hamish seemed hungry, Heidi would order ham sandwiches for him. At the end of the holiday, Heidi put her hamster back into her suitcase. Heather's mother did wonder why there were holes in her hamper, but Heather and Heidi did not tell her.

Puzzle worksheet for the 'h' sound

Use the 'h' pictures to help you with these puzzles.

Unscramble the words below. They all begin with 'h'.

1 tha   **2** enh   **3** ndha   **4** ehosr   **5** mhmrea

_____   _____   _____   _____   _____

Look for the 'h' words in the wordsearch below. They can
read down or across. There are eight 'h' words of three or
more letters.

o	y	r	h	e	e	l	w
q	e	t	o	u	s	f	g
j	h	m	s	k	h	a	t
h	e	n	p	z	c	b	m
o	a	v	i	h	a	n	d
r	d	c	t	z	w	q	r
s	y	h	a	i	r	f	k
e	v	d	l	p	y	s	z

Write down the words that you found:

1 _____   2 _____

3 _____   4 _____

5 _____   6 _____

7 _____   8 _____

Illustrations for the 'h' sound

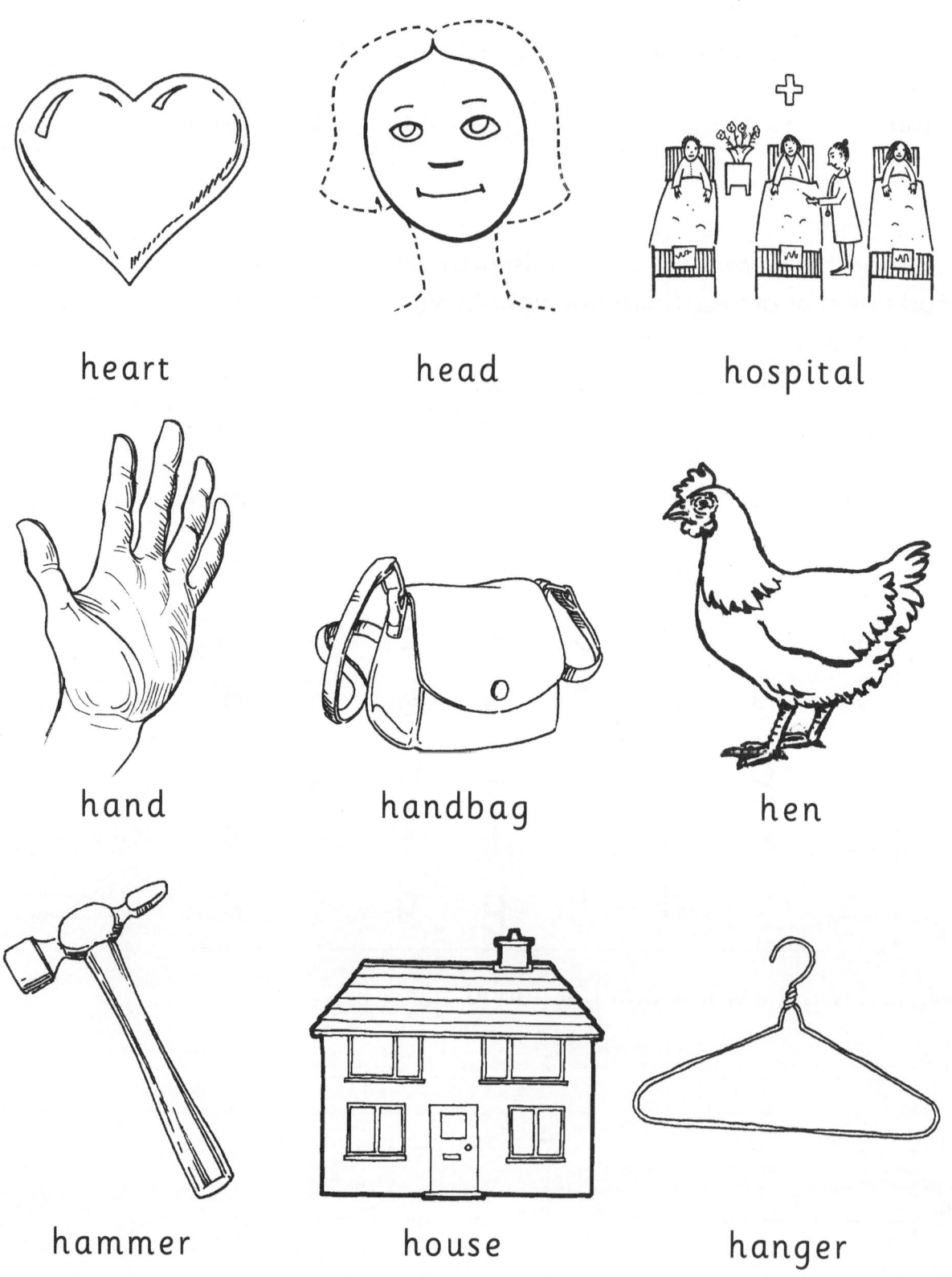

heart

head

hospital

hand

handbag

hen

hammer

house

hanger

Illustrations for the 'h' sound

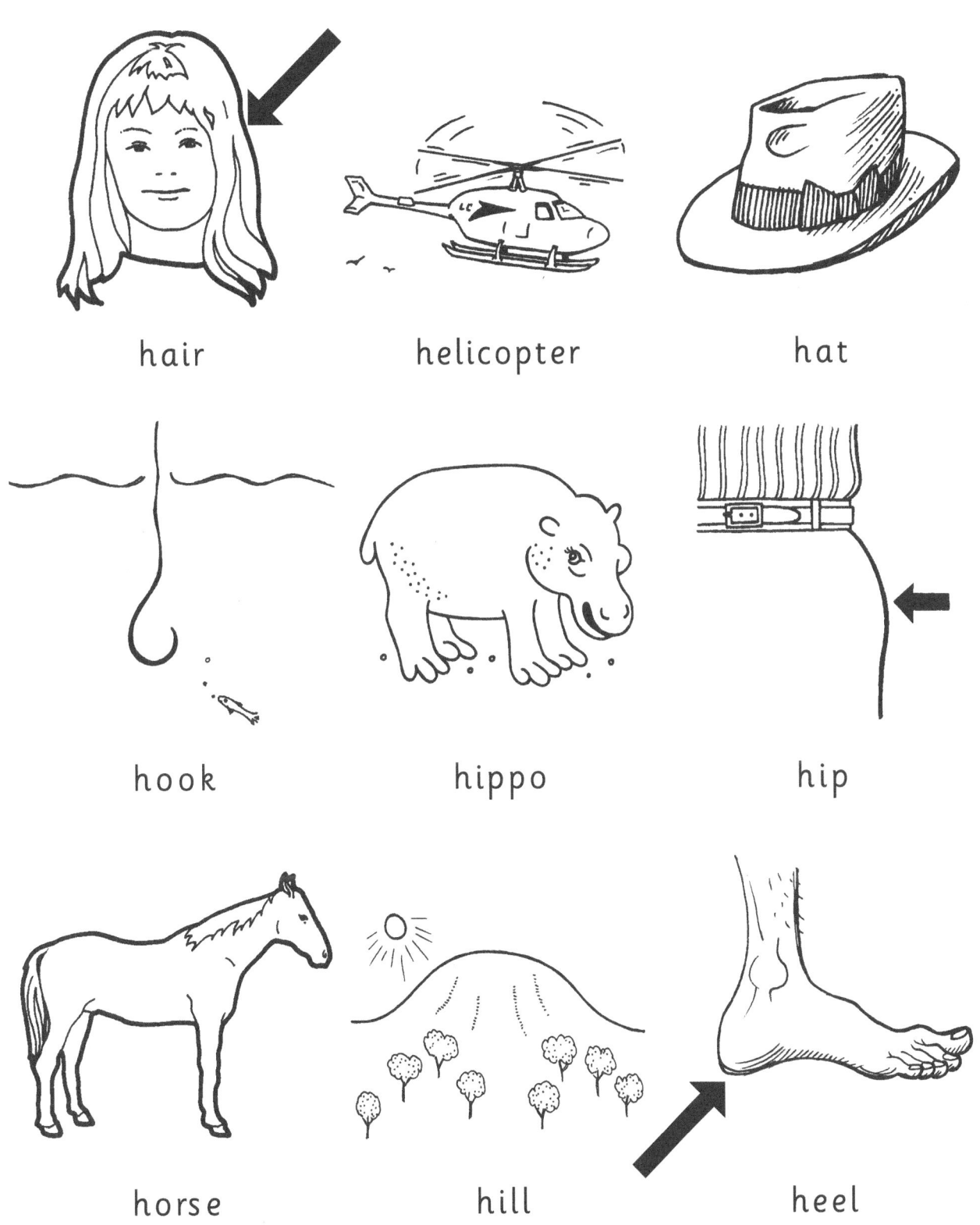

hair

helicopter

hat

hook

hippo

hip

horse

hill

heel

2/2

Section for the 'j' sound

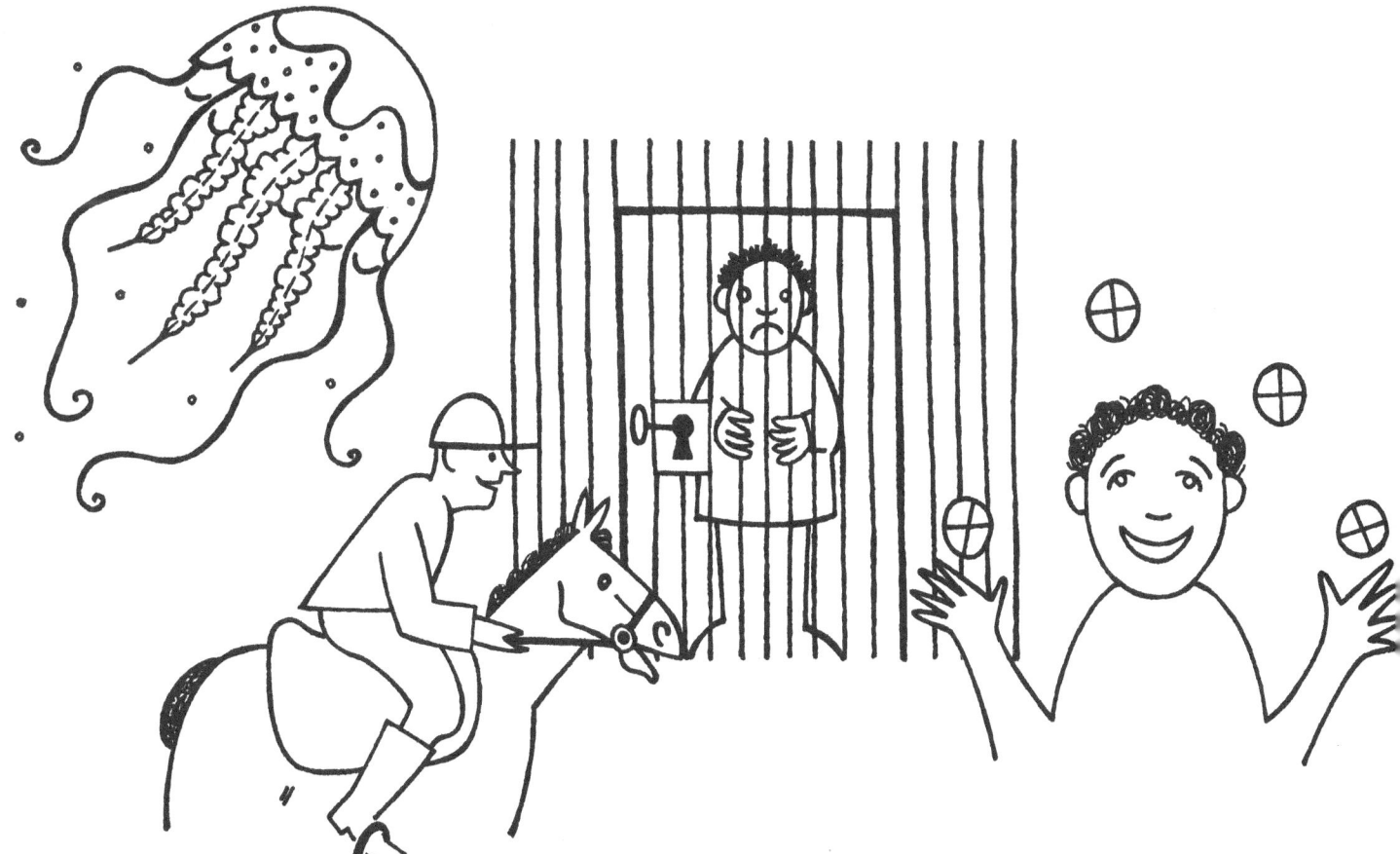

Section for the 'j' sound

Riddles for the 'j' sound

→ Children are given the photocopied pictures to go with the target sound. The teacher reads out the riddles, one at a time, and the children decide which picture each one refers to. If desired, the children can then colour these pictures in.

→ *To make the activity more difficult*, the children, without access to the pictures, are told the target sound, and the riddles are read out one at a time. The children have to think of something that starts with that sound and fits in with the riddle.

→ *To teach vocabulary*, the teacher and the children look together at the photocopied pictures, and the teacher names and talks about each illustration. The teacher then proceeds to read out the riddles as suggested above.

1 This lives in the sea. It might sting you. (*jellyfish*)
2 These are usually blue. They are like trousers. (*jeans*)
3 This has sleeves and buttons or a zip. You could wear it over a jumper. (*jacket*)
4 You can eat this. It could be green, orange, red or yellow. (*jelly*)
5 It has a handle. You might put milk in it. (*jug*)
6 This can go fast. It flies in the sky. (*jet*)
7 This comes from oranges or apples. You drink it. (*juice*)
8 It is sticky. You put it on bread. (*jam*)
9 He takes part in a race. He rides a horse. (*jockey*)
10 This is worn when it is cold. It does not have zips or buttons. (*jumper*)
11 He might work in a circus. He throws things into the air. (*juggler*)
12 This is a part of your face. It is below your nose. (*jaw*)

Alliteration for the 'j' sound

Suitable for children in Years R, 1 and 2

→ The teacher states what the target sound is. They then read out each two-word phrase, and, after each one, the children must say whether one word or both words start with the target sound.

→ Alternatively, the teacher can give each child two cards with the target sound printed on. If both words in the phrase begin with the target sound, the children hold up two cards. If only one begins with that sound, they hold up one card.

strawberry jam	juicy orange
jealous jockey	green jelly
milk jug	jam jar
woolly jumper	fast jet
jolly juggler	wooden jigsaw
jumping jellyfish	dangerous jungle

Tongue twisters for the 'j' sound

Suitable for children in Years R, 1 and 2

→ The teacher reads each tongue twister aloud and, after each one, asks the children to repeat it once or twice.

→ The children can play a game of Chinese Whispers. The teacher whispers the tongue twister to one child; this child whispers it to the next and so on. The last child says out loud what they think the teacher said, and this is compared with the original tongue twister.

1 Jealous Jean jumped for joy.
2 Jacob and Jasmin joined Jim in the jungle.
3 The judge joined Jack, the jockey, for the journey.
4 Joe, the jolly juggler, juggled with the jars of jam.
5 John jogged from Jamestown to Jacksonville.

Odd word out — initial sounds

Involving words beginning with the 'j' sound

→ The children are told which initial sound to listen for. They then listen
while the teacher reads aloud one line of three words at a time. After
each line the children are asked to say which word did not begin with
the target sound.

1	jug	jar	dog
2	jail	well	jaw
3	jump	jog	match
4	June	cone	job
5	ball	jet	jam
6	jeans	chair	juice
7	chick	Jack	joint
8	judge	join	dodge
9	mist	just	junk
10	July	shiny	journey
11	jumper	lemon	jelly
12	table	jockey	jacket
13	jolly	jealous	smelly
14	jigsaw	bumper	juggler
15	joker	jungle	finger

Odd word out – rhyming
Using a word beginning with the 'j' sound

→ The children are told to listen for the word that does not rhyme with the other two. They then listen while the teacher reads aloud one line of three words at a time. After each line the children are asked to say which word does not rhyme with the other two.

→ Alternatively, the children could be asked to say which two words do rhyme.

→ As an extra task, the children could think of other words that rhyme with the two rhyming words in each set.

1	jaw	sea	four
2	jug	mug	gum
3	sat	jet	wet
4	jar	car	tie
5	jail	chain	tail
6	doors	jeans	beans
7	jam	bat	ham
8	jacket	wicket	packet
9	hamper	jumper	bumper
10	jelly	silly	smelly

Words to sound out for the 'j' sound

→ Only words with regular spelling have been included.

→ The teacher takes one word at a time and 'sounds out' each phoneme. This may need to be done several times. The children must then guess what the word is. Some children may be able to try writing the word.

→ The children may like to repeat the phonemes consecutively, just as the teacher did, to help them blend the sounds into words.

j—a—m	j—u—g	j—ar	j—e—t
j—ai—l	j—u—m—p	j—o—g	j—oi—n

Story for the 'j' sound

→ The teacher asks the children to listen carefully to the story and pick out the words beginning with the target sound. The teacher then reads the story, sentence by sentence. After each sentence the teacher asks the children:
  – To say how many words they heard beginning with the given sound in that sentence.
  – To repeat the words they heard beginning with the target sound.
→ Alternatively, the teacher can slowly read the whole story, and the children can make a tally mark on a piece of paper every time they hear a word beginning with the target sound. The children can then count up how many words they have heard beginning with that sound and tell the teacher what those words are.

The horse race

It was 21st January and Jake and Jill were going to watch their dad riding. Mr Jolly, their dad, was a jockey. His horse was called Jellybeans. It was a cold day, so Jake, Jill and Mrs Jolly put on their thick jumpers and denim jackets and jeans for their journey to the race course. On the way there, they got caught up in a traffic jam. Jake and Jill were so thirsty that they drank a whole jug of orange juice between them. Finally Jill, Jake and Mrs Jolly arrived at the race course. Mr Jolly was already riding Jellybeans to the start. Jill looked at the fences that Jellybeans would have to jump over. All the jockeys were ready, and the horses were off. Jake and Jill jumped up and down with excitement. Jellybeans jumped all the fences easily, but Joker, the grey horse, was in front. Jellybeans and Joker raced to the finishing line. Jellybeans just beat Joker by a nose. Jake, Jill and Mrs Jolly jumped for joy.

Puzzle worksheet for the 'j' sound

Use the 'j' pictures to help you with these puzzles.

Unscramble the words below. They all begin with 'j'.

1 ugj   **2** wja   **3** leyjl   **4** okjyce   **5** umepjr

_____   _____   _____   _____   _____

Look for the 'j' words in the wordsearch below. They can read down or across. There are eight 'j' words of three letters or more.

v	j	g	j	e	l	l	y
j	u	g	y	r	f	c	x
s	g	w	q	a	j	z	j
m	g	p	k	j	e	n	o
j	l	y	j	a	m	h	c
b	e	v	e	w	p	f	k
q	r	w	t	v	e	k	e
j	u	i	c	e	r	n	y

Write down the words that you found:

1 _____   2 _____

3 _____   4 _____

5 _____   6 _____

7 _____   8 _____

73

Illustrations for the 'j' sound

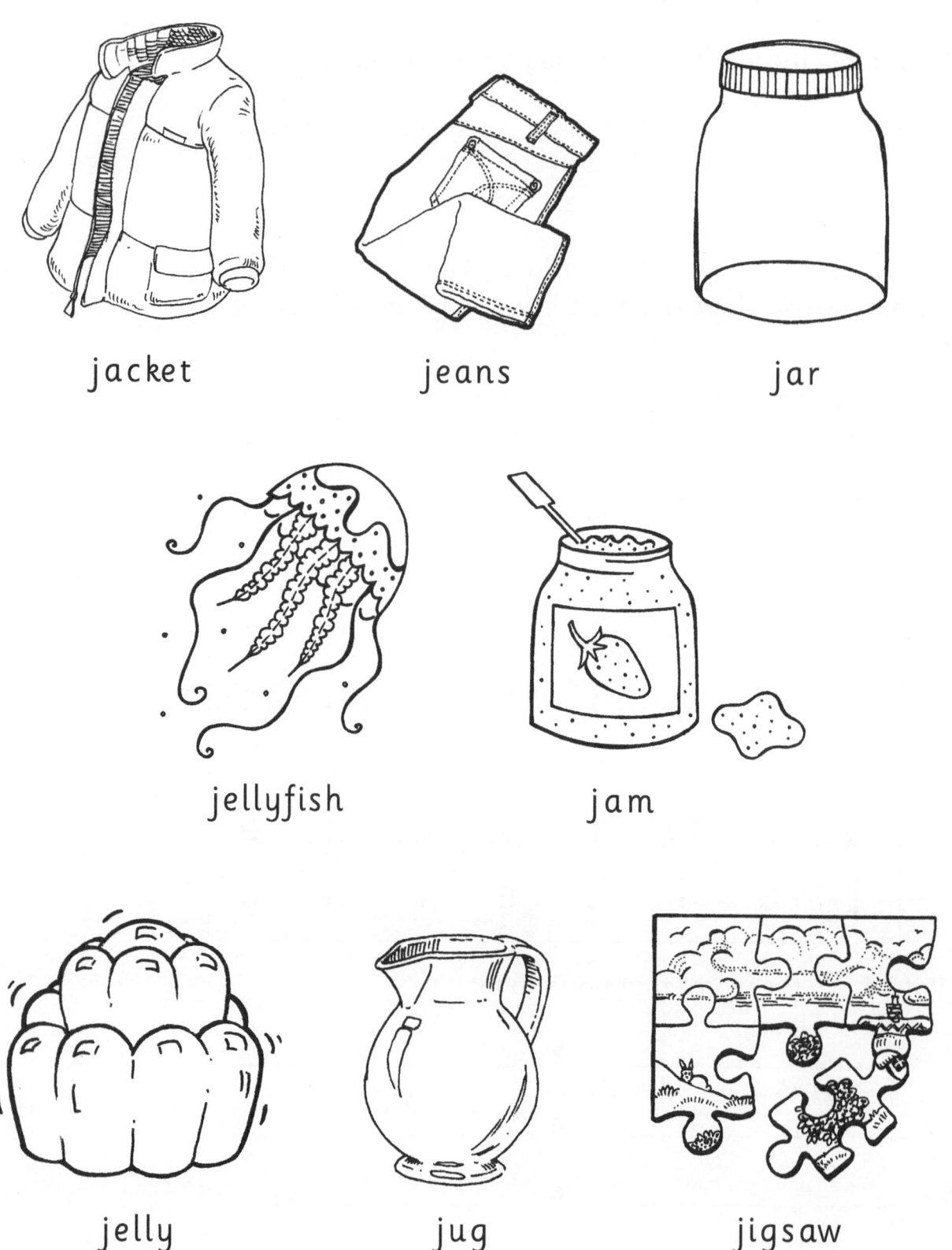

jacket

jeans

jar

jellyfish

jam

jelly

jug

jigsaw

Illustrations for the 'j' sound

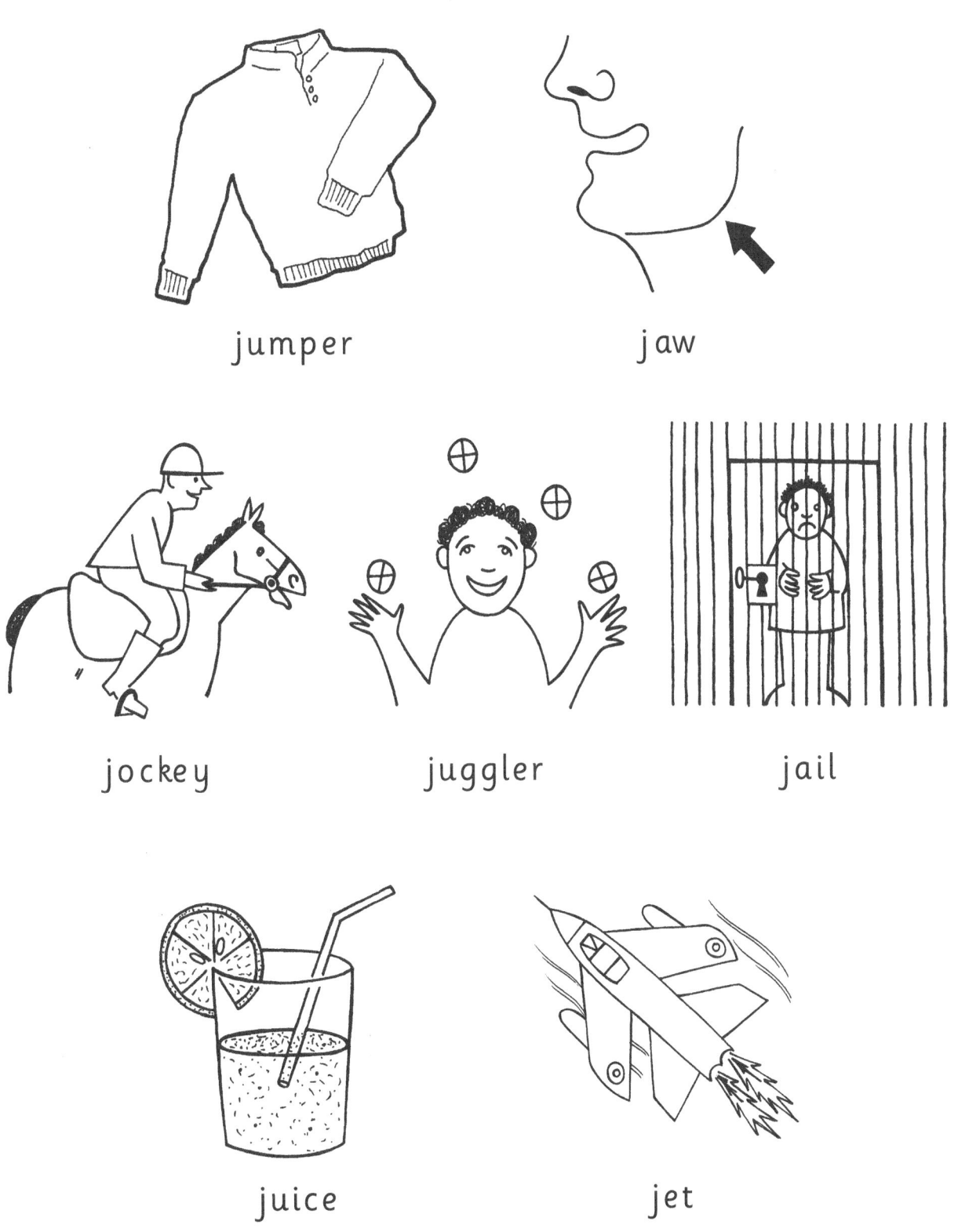

jumper

jaw

jockey

juggler

jail

juice

jet

2/2

Section for the 'l' sound

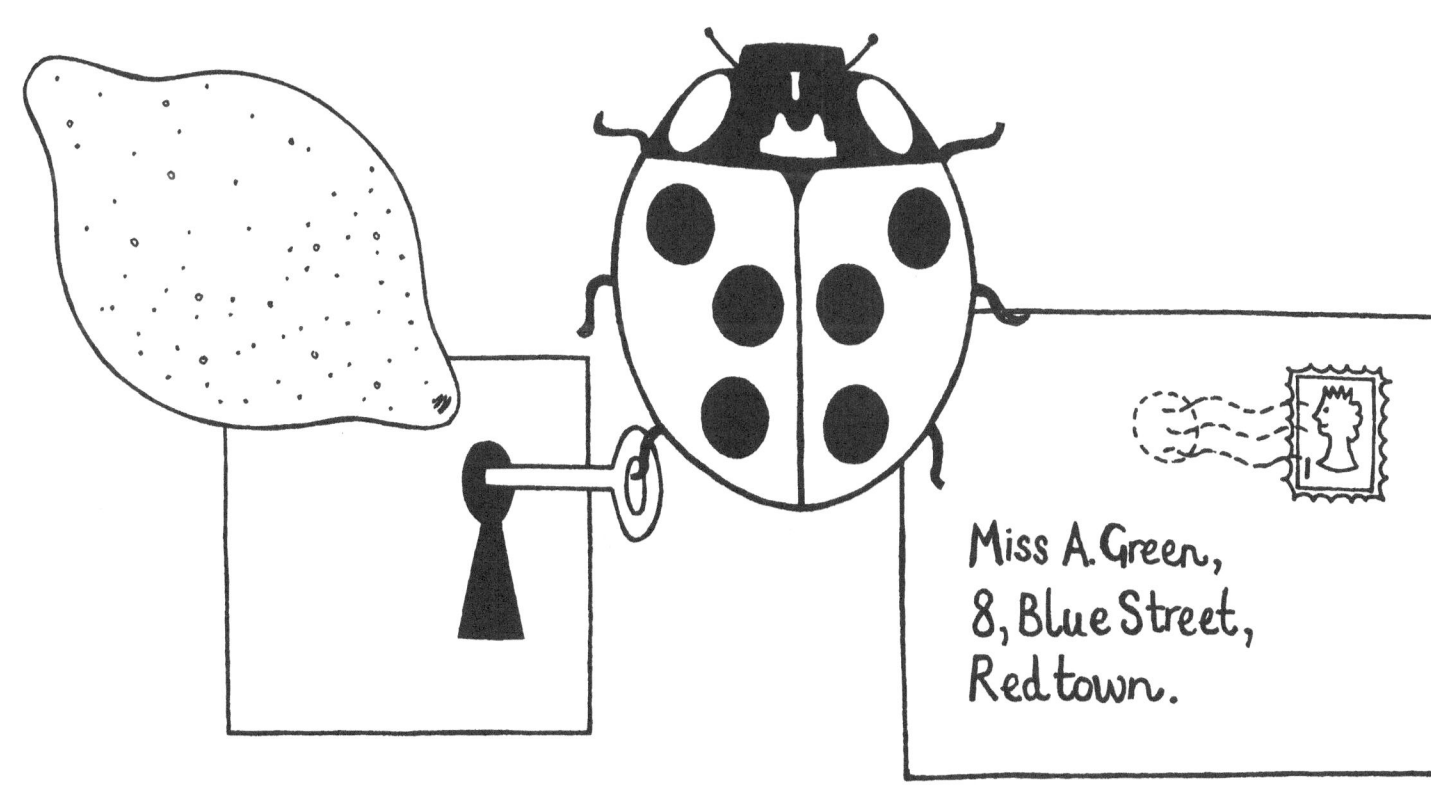

Miss A. Green,
8, Blue Street,
Redtown.

Section for the 'l' sound

Riddles for the 'l' sound

→ Children are given the photocopied pictures to go with the target sound. The teacher reads out the riddles, one at a time, and the children decide which picture each one refers to. If desired, the children can then colour these pictures in.

→ *To make the activity more difficult*, the children, without access to the pictures, are told the target sound, and the riddles are read out one at a time. The children have to think of something that starts with that sound and fits in with the riddle.

→ *To teach vocabulary*, the teacher and the children look together at the photocopied pictures, and the teacher names and talks about each illustration. The teacher then proceeds to read out the riddles as suggested above.

1   It might be green, yellow, red or brown. It might fall off a tree in autumn. (*leaf*)
2   They are part of your face. They are part of your mouth. (*lips*)
3   It has a mane. It has sharp teeth and claws. (*lion*)
4   It is yellow. It tastes sour. (*lemon*)
5   Its father is a ram. Its mother is a ewe. (*lamb*)
6   It has a stamp on it. You post it. (*letter*)
7   It has a light. The light flashes on and off. (*lighthouse*)
8   It has rungs. You can climb it. (*ladder*)
9   You can switch it off and on. It has a bulb and a shade on it. (*lamp*)
10   It is part of your body. It is between your hip and your foot. (*leg*)
11   This is made of metal. It has a keyhole. (*lock*)
12   It carries heavy loads. It has wheels. (*lorry*)

Alliteration for the 'l' sound

→ The teacher states what the target sound is. They then read out each two-word phrase, and, after each one, the children must say whether one word or both words start with the target sound.

→ Alternatively, the teacher can give each child two cards with the target sound printed on. If both words in the phrase begin with the target sound, the children hold up two cards. If only one begins with that sound, they hold up one card.

lovely lady	low wall
little lamb	long ladder
short legs	large lorry
red lips	loud noise
lucky ladybird	lazy lion
juicy lemon	lonely lizard

Tongue twisters for the 'l' sound

→ The teacher reads each tongue twister aloud and, after each one, asks the children to repeat it once or twice.

→ The children can play a game of Chinese Whispers. The teacher whispers the tongue twister to one child; this child whispers it to the next and so on. The last child says out loud what they think the teacher said, and this is compared with the original tongue twister.

1 The lazy leopard laughed at the little ladybird.
2 Libby licked the lovely lime and lemon lollipop.
3 Larry the lamb limped down the long lane.
4 Louis liked to leap off long ladders and land on the lawn.
5 Leo left the luscious lobster in the laundry.

Odd word out – initial sounds

Involving words beginning with the 'l' sound

→ The children are told which initial sound to listen for. They then listen while the teacher reads aloud one line of three words at a time. After each line the children are asked to say which word did not begin with the target sound.

1	lamp	man	like
2	rain	look	loud
3	live	leaf	push
4	run	long	left
5	leg	lake	tug
6	lid	pill	laugh
7	lime	loaf	nail
8	stop	love	lap
9	lips	sack	lock
10	lost	log	owl
11	large	back	lane
12	ladder	collar	lorry
13	tractor	letter	lazy
14	lettuce	rocket	lizard
15	ladybird	leopard	fairy

Odd word out – rhyming
Using a word beginning with the 'l' sound

➜ The children are told to listen for the word that does not rhyme with the other two. They then listen while the teacher reads aloud one line of three words at a time. After each line the children are asked to say which word does not rhyme with the other two.

➜ Alternatively, the children could be asked to say which two words do rhyme.

➜ As an extra task, the children could think of other words that rhyme with the two rhyming words in each set.

1	lid	hid	pod
2	grass	lock	flock
3	lips	mops	hips
4	bump	camp	lamp
5	leg	peg	bag
6	cough	laugh	half
7	lime	time	same
8	lizard	buzzer	wizard
9	merry	lorry	sorry
10	letter	better	fitter

Words to sound out for the 'l' sound

➜ Only words with regular spelling have been included.

➜ The teacher takes one word at a time and 'sounds out' each phoneme. This may need to be done several times. The children must then guess what the word is. Some children may be able to try writing the word.

➜ The children may like to repeat the phonemes consecutively, just as the teacher did, to help them blend the sounds into words.

l—e—g	l—i—d	l—o—ck	l—o—g
l—a—m—p	l—oa—f	l—i—p	l—ea—f

Story for the 'l' sound

→ The teacher asks the children to listen carefully to the story and pick out the words beginning with the target sound. The teacher then reads the story, sentence by sentence. After each sentence the teacher asks the children:

- To say how many words they heard beginning with the given sound in that sentence.
- To repeat the words they heard beginning with the target sound.

→ Alternatively, the teacher can slowly read the whole story, and the children can make a tally mark on a piece of paper every time they hear a word beginning with the target sound. The children can then count up how many words they have heard beginning with that sound and tell the teacher what those words are.

Lucky the lamb

Lucy and Leon, her elder brother, had a pet lamb called Lucky. When Lucky was born, his leg was twisted and he became lame. One day, Lucy asked Leon to walk up the hill to Lucky's field with her. Leon said that he had a letter to write. It was an excuse because Leon was lazy and did not like walking. Lucy took a packed lunch with her. She sat down and watched Lucky leaping around on his lame leg. Then Lucy lay down on the long green grass and fell asleep. Meanwhile, the sky began to look very black. A loud clap of thunder woke Lucy up. Lucy ran to shelter under an old lime tree. A streak of lightning struck the lime tree, and a log, which had been leaning against it, fell on Lucy. Leon was worried because it was late and his sister Lucy had been gone for a long time. Leon decided to go and look for Lucy. Walking up the hill, Leon heard Lucky bleating loudly. Leon followed the sound. Looking through the lashing rain, he saw Lucy. Lucy's leg was trapped by the log. Leon carefully lifted the log off Lucy's leg. Then he lifted Lucy onto his shoulder and carried her home, with Lucky leading the way.

Puzzle worksheet for the 'l' sound

Use the 'l' pictures to help you with these puzzles.

Unscramble the words below. They all begin with 'l'.

1 egl   **2** glo   **3** mpla   **4** ilno   **5** mneol

_____   _____   _____   _____   _____

Look for the 'l' words in the wordsearch below. They can read down or across. There are eight 'l' words of three letters or more.

l	a	d	d	e	r	z	m
a	s	k	q	l	o	g	l
d	p	x	l	j	d	r	e
y	e	l	i	o	n	y	t
b	t	v	d	j	l	p	t
i	h	f	w	e	i	n	u
r	o	l	a	m	p	u	c
d	x	c	q	b	s	z	e

Write down the words that you found:

1 _____   **2** _____

3 _____   **4** _____

5 _____   **6** _____

7 _____   **8** _____

83

Illustrations for the 'l' sound

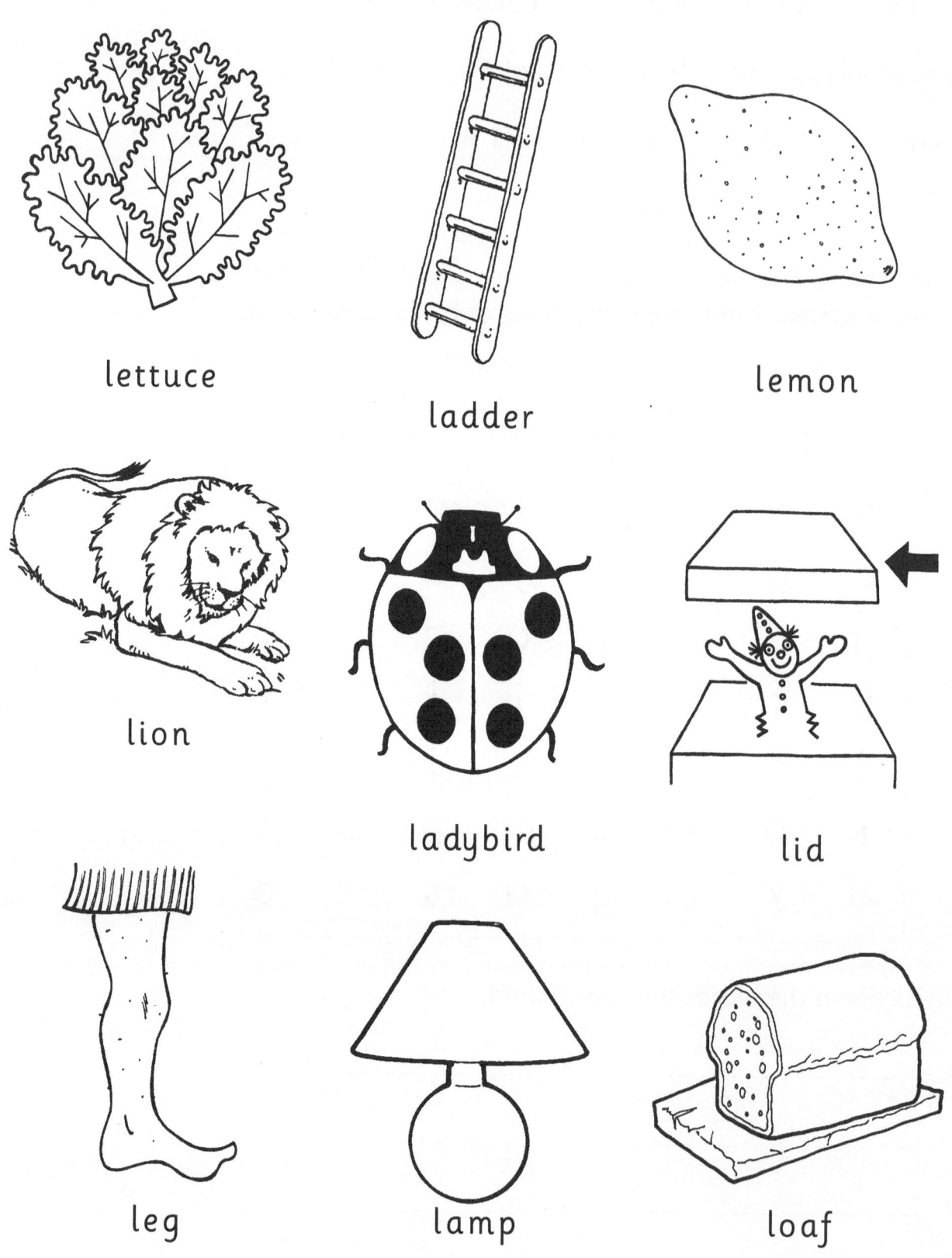

lettuce

ladder

lemon

lion

ladybird

lid

leg

lamp

loaf

Illustrations for the 'l' sound

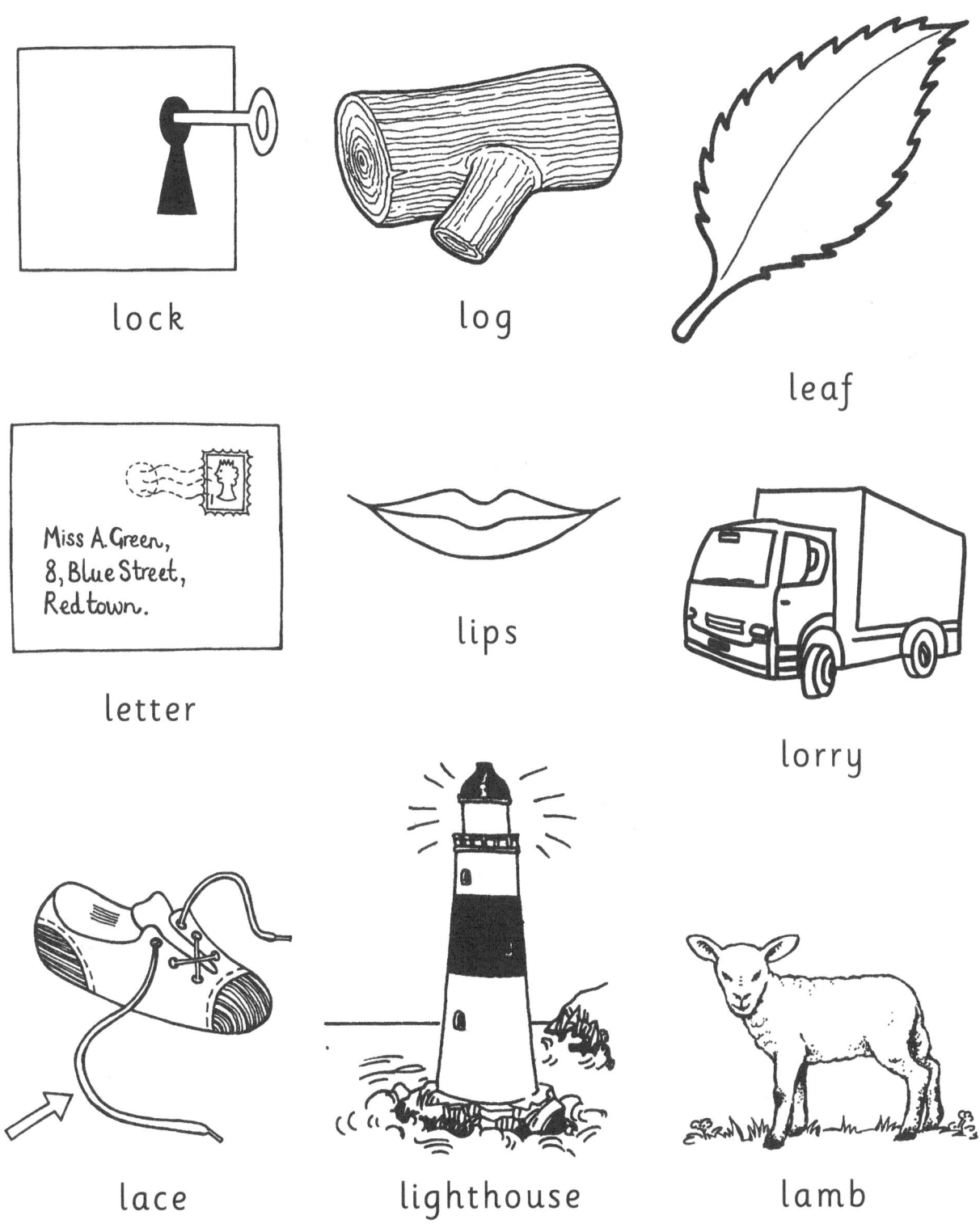

lock

log

leaf

letter

Miss A. Green,
8, Blue Street,
Redtown.

lips

lorry

lace

lighthouse

lamb

2/2

Section for the 'm' sound

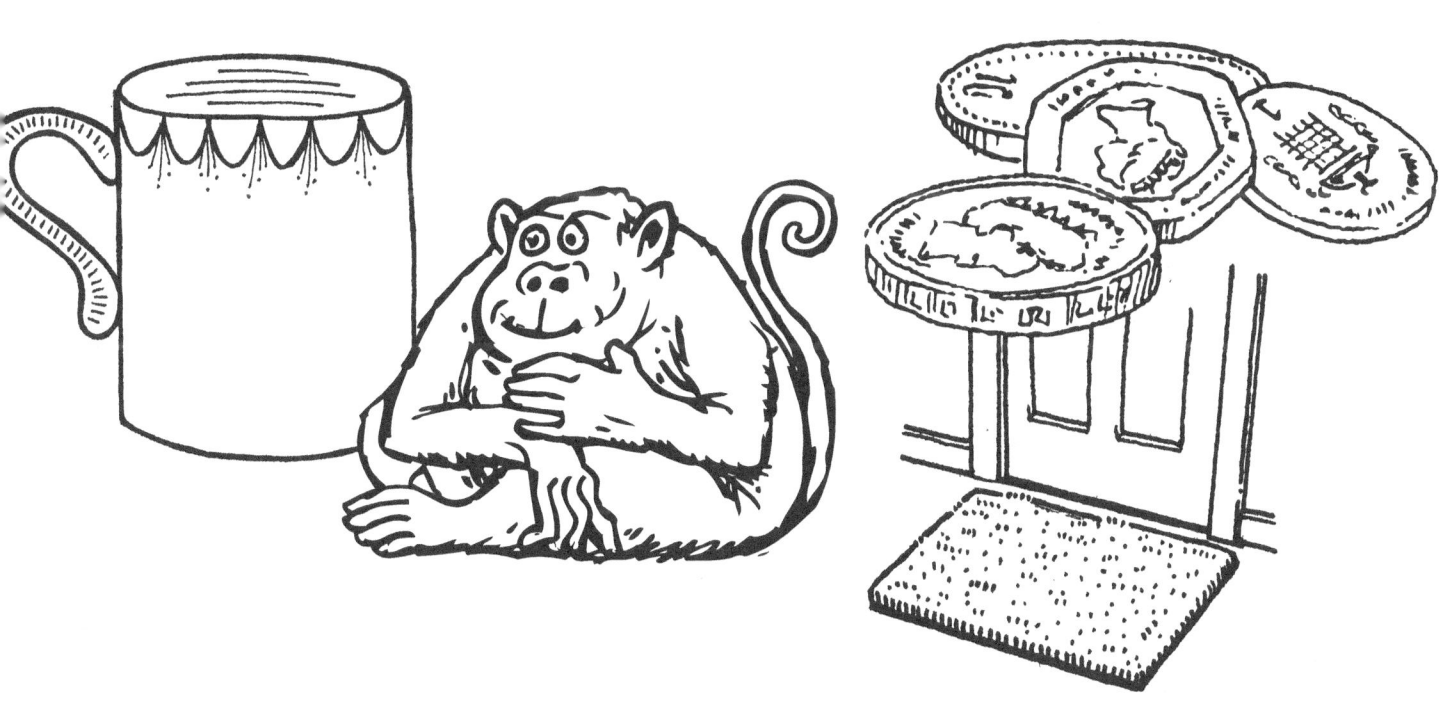

Section for the 'm' sound

Suitable for children in Year R

Riddles for the 'm' sound

→ Children are given the photocopied pictures to go with the target sound. The teacher reads out the riddles, one at a time, and the children decide which picture each one refers to. If desired, the children can then colour these pictures in.

→ *To make the activity more difficult*, the children, without access to the pictures, are told the target sound, and the riddles are read out one at a time. The children have to think of something that starts with that sound and fits in with the riddle.

→ *To teach vocabulary*, the teacher and the children look together at the photocopied pictures, and the teacher names and talks about each illustration. The teacher then proceeds to read out the riddles as suggested above.

1   You might put this in tea or coffee. It comes from a cow. (*milk*)
2   You eat this. You can buy it from the butcher's. (*meat*)
3   It is an animal. It can swing from tree to tree. (*monkey*)
4   It has a handle. You wash the floor with it. (*mop*)
5   It is made from oranges. You might spread it on toast. (*marmalade*)
6   It is made from glass. You can see yourself in it. (*mirror*)
7   It is very high. Some people climb up it. (*mountain*)
8   It has a thumb but no fingers. You wear it when it is cold. (*mitten*)
9   It has a handle. You drink out of it. (*mug*)
10   Sometimes you see all of it in the sky. Sometimes you only see part of it. (*moon*)
11   It is part of your body. You put food into it. (*mouth*)
12   It is a small animal. It does not like cats. (*mouse*)

Alliteration for the 'm' sound

→ The teacher states what the target sound is. They then read out each two-word phrase, and, after each one, the children must say whether one word or both words start with the target sound.

→ Alternatively, the teacher can give each child two cards with the target sound printed on. If both words in the phrase begin with the target sound, the children hold up two cards. If only one begins with that sound, they hold up one card.

messy monkey	tiny mouse
muddy mittens	merry monster
mad donkey	lazy mice
magic mirror	ripe melon
mucky mop	many mugs
dirty motorbike	raw meat

Tongue twisters for the 'm' sound

→ The teacher reads each tongue twister aloud and, after each one, asks the children to repeat it once or twice.

→ The children can play a game of Chinese Whispers. The teacher whispers the tongue twister to one child; this child whispers it to the next and so on. The last child says out loud what they think the teacher said, and this is compared with the original tongue twister.

1 Maddison married Mark in Madrid.
2 Mike moored his motorboat at Margate.
3 The metal monster made a muddy mess.
4 Magda's mother made mushroom and mustard muffins.
5 The magician made more marmalade meringues.

Odd word out — initial sounds

Involving words beginning with the 'm' sound

→ The children are told which initial sound to listen for. They then listen while the teacher reads aloud one line of three words at a time. After each line the children are asked to say which word did not begin with the target sound.

1	mug	mask	knock
2	mop	can	milk
3	bat	man	mouse
4	meat	fan	map
5	vet	moon	mouth
6	mud	dull	mat
7	moth	met	lamb
8	mum	mad	bed
9	mill	hall	mole
10	bend	mast	men
11	money	mirror	pretty
12	noodle	middle	metal
13	monkey	donkey	mitten
14	mountain	measure	beaver
15	piano	medal	mechanic

Odd word out — rhyming

Using a word beginning with the 'm' sound

Suitable for children in Years R, 1 and 2

→ The children are told to listen for the word that does not rhyme with the other two. They then listen while the teacher reads aloud one line of three words at a time. After each line the children are asked to say which word does not rhyme with the other two.

→ Alternatively, the children could be asked to say which two words do rhyme.

→ As an extra task, the children could think of other words that rhyme with the two rhyming words in each set.

1	map	ten	cap
2	mole	hole	pin
3	meat	dog	seat
4	swim	man	can
5	mug	dug	jam
6	milk	walk	silk
7	face	mouse	house
8	mouth	north	south
9	money	sandy	honey
10	metal	petal	bottle

Words to sound out for the 'm' sound

Suitable for children in Years R, 1 and 2

→ Only words with regular spelling have been included.

→ The teacher takes one word at a time and 'sounds out' each phoneme. This may need to be done several times. The children must then guess what the word is. Some children may be able to try writing the word.

→ The children may like to repeat the phonemes consecutively, just as the teacher did, to help them blend the sounds into words.

m—u—g	m—o—p	m—a—n	m—ea—t
m—a—p	m—a—t	m—oo—n	m—ou—th

Story for the 'm' sound

→ The teacher asks the children to listen carefully to the story and pick out the words beginning with the target sound. The teacher then reads the story, sentence by sentence. After each sentence the teacher asks the children:
  - To say how many words they heard beginning with the given sound in that sentence.
  - To repeat the words they heard beginning with the target sound.
→ Alternatively, the teacher can slowly read the whole story, and the children can make a tally mark on a piece of paper every time they hear a word beginning with the target sound. The children can then count up how many words they have heard beginning with that sound and tell the teacher what those words are.

The mischievous monkey

Megan had a mischievous monkey called Mickey. One day Megan decided to make some melon mousse. Mickey sat on the mat merrily munching some mangoes and some marmalade sandwiches. Megan went to the fridge and got out some cream and a melon. She put the cream and the melon into a mixing bowl and mixed them together. Megan looked through the window and saw her mate Martha coming up the path. She went outside to meet Martha. Meanwhile, the mischievous monkey had climbed onto the table and tipped the melon mixture all over himself. He then marched along the kitchen work surface, knocking off a jar of mustard and making a terrible mess. When Megan came back and saw the mess, she was not very pleased. She told the mischievous monkey that he would have to go without his supper of mashed bananas and milk.

Routledge Taylor & Francis Group

Puzzle worksheet for the 'm' sound

Use the 'm' pictures to help you with these puzzles.

Unscramble the words below. They all begin with 'm'.

1 mpo   **2** gmu   **3** lkmi   **4** emta   **5** nmyoe

_____   _____   _____   _____   _____

Look for the 'm' words in the wordsearch below. They can read down or across. There are eight 'm' words of three letters or more.

p	m	u	g	l	k	j	n
h	o	b	o	g	m	v	c
d	u	r	m	f	o	t	y
v	n	m	o	o	n	b	m
y	t	q	n	x	k	b	a
m	a	p	e	p	e	s	n
z	i	j	y	h	y	v	d
g	n	w	m	o	u	s	e

Write down the words that you found:

1 _____   2 _____

3 _____   4 _____

5 _____   6 _____

7 _____   8 _____

93

Illustrations for the 'm' sound

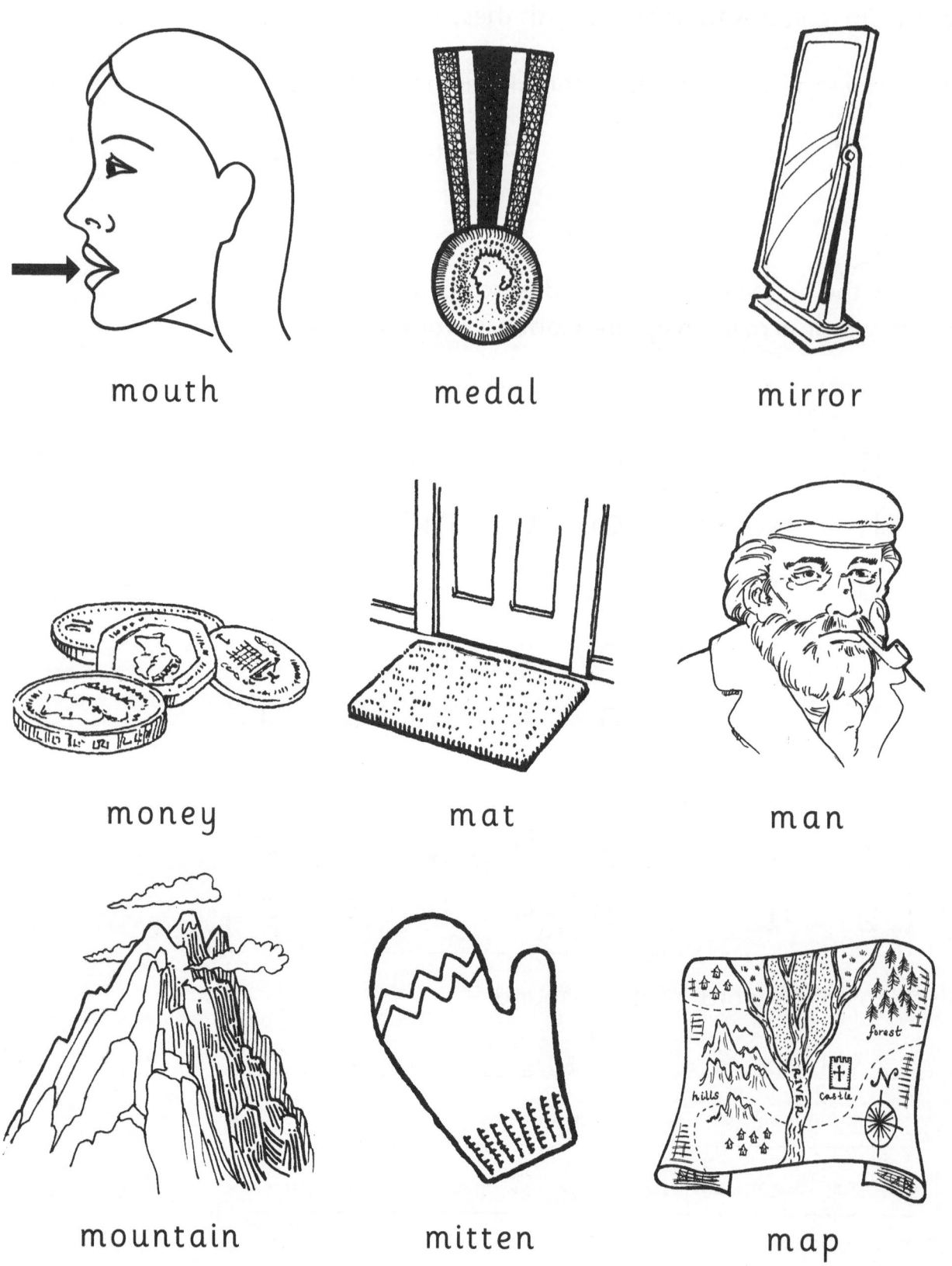

mouth

medal

mirror

money

mat

man

mountain

mitten

map

Illustrations for the 'm' sound

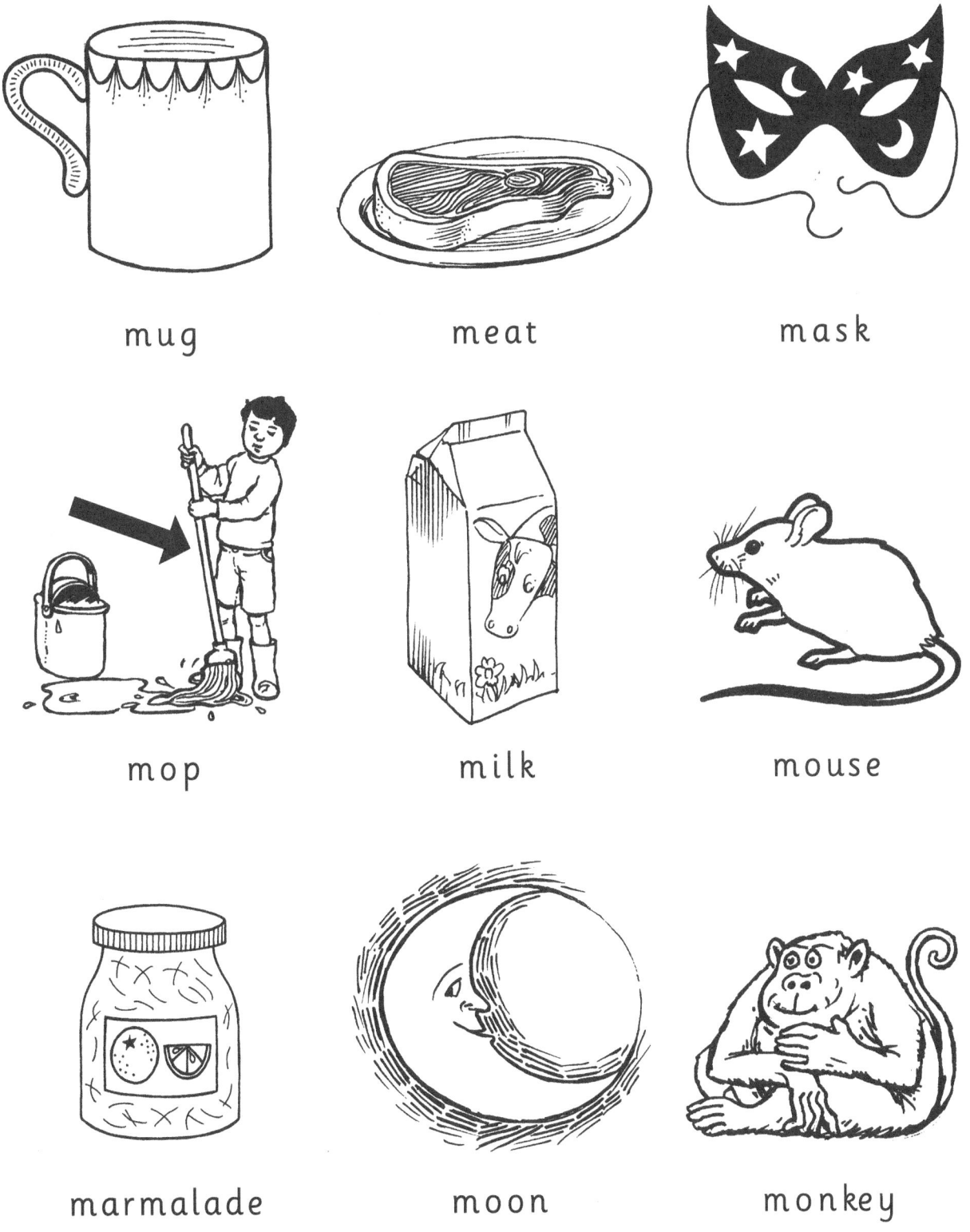

mug

meat

mask

mop

milk

mouse

marmalade

moon

monkey

2/2

Section for the 'n' sound

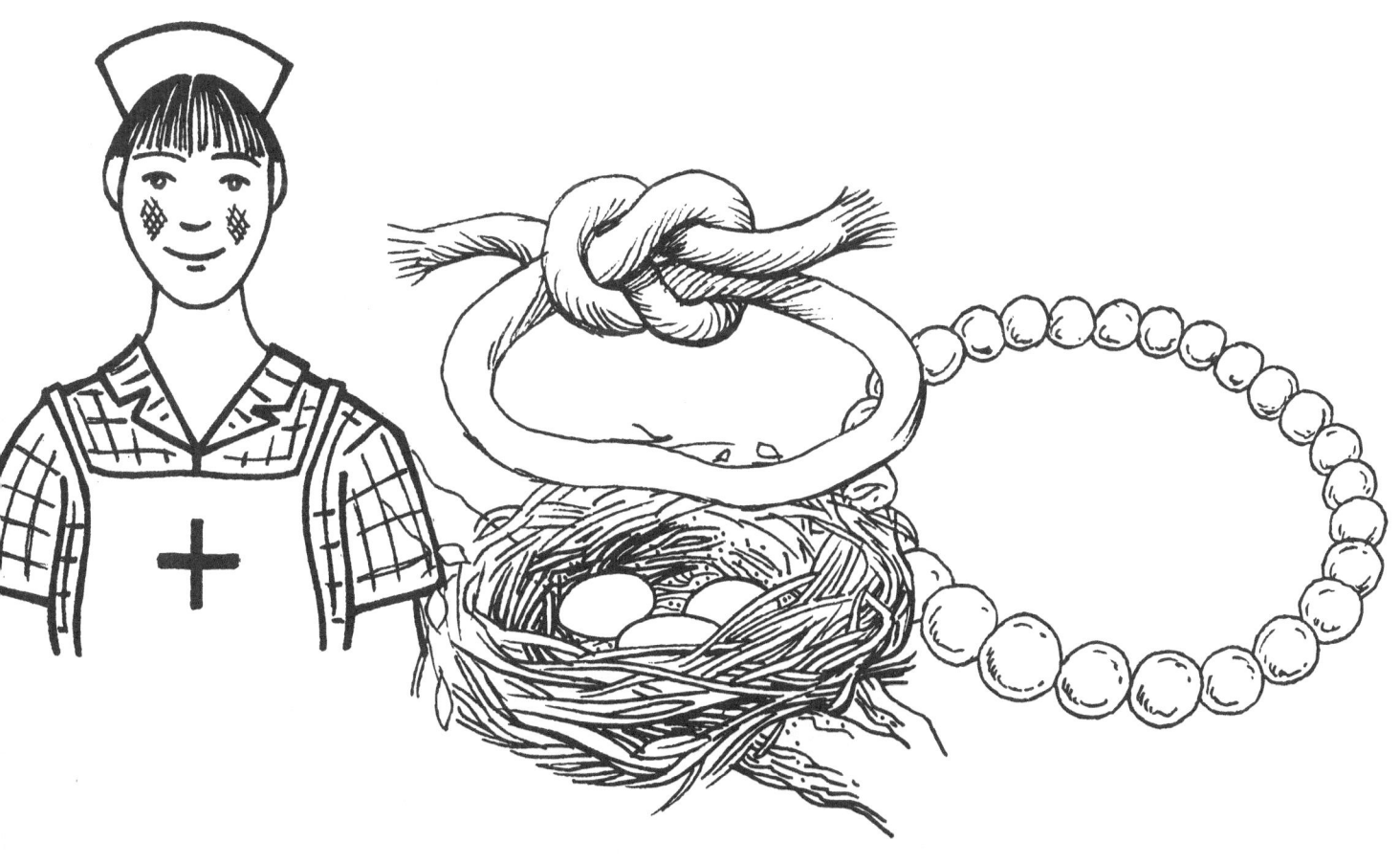

Section for the 'n' sound

Riddles for the 'n' sound

→ Children are given the photocopied pictures to go with the target sound. The teacher reads out the riddles, one at a time, and the children decide which picture each one refers to. If desired, the children can then colour these pictures in.

→ *To make the activity more difficult*, the children, without access to the pictures, are told the target sound, and the riddles are read out one at a time. The children have to think of something that starts with that sound and fits in with the riddle.

→ *To teach vocabulary*, the teacher and the children look together at the photocopied pictures, and the teacher names and talks about each illustration. The teacher then proceeds to read out the riddles as suggested above.

1   It is made of metal. You use a hammer on it. (*nail*)
2   It is pretty. You put it round your neck. (*necklace*)
3   Everyone has one. It might be Sanjay, Amy or Louis. (*name*)
4   It is made of metal. It has an eye. (*needle*)
5   It is made of twigs, moss and grass. It might have eggs in it. (*nest*)
6   You can eat it. It has a shell. (*nut*)
7   This is someone who wears a uniform. They look after sick people. (*nurse*)
8   This is part of your body. It has two nostrils. (*nose*)
9   It has lots of holes in it. You might catch fish with it. (*net*)
10 It has a handle. You use it to eat with. (*knife*)
11 It is part of your body. It is in the middle of your leg. (*knee*)
12 Most of it is black and white. You can read it. (*newspaper*)

Alliteration for the 'n' sound

Suitable for children in Years R, 1 and 2

→ The teacher states what the target sound is. They then read out each two-word phrase, and, after each one, the children must say whether one word or both words start with the target sound.

→ Alternatively, the teacher can give each child two cards with the target sound printed on. If both words in the phrase begin with the target sound, the children hold up two cards. If only one begins with that sound, they hold up one card.

noisy nurse	naughty chimp
dark night	nice nut
filthy nose	soft nightie
narrow neck	nasty nettle
sharp nail	nine nests
daily newspaper	knobbly knees

Tongue twisters for the 'n' sound

Suitable for children in Years R, 1 and 2

→ The teacher reads each tongue twister aloud and, after each one, asks the children to repeat it once or twice.

→ The children can play a game of Chinese Whispers. The teacher whispers the tongue twister to one child; this child whispers it to the next and so on. The last child says out loud what they think the teacher said, and this is compared with the original tongue twister.

1 Nina needed nine knitting needles.
2 Nigel's nanny knocked her knee on the knob.
3 Neither Niall nor Norman knew the number of knives needed.
4 Nancy noticed her nephew knocking nails in the gnome's nose.
5 Nick's noisy neighbour's name was Nadine.

Odd word out — initial sounds

Involving words beginning with the 'n' sound

→ The children are told which initial sound to listen for. They then listen while the teacher reads aloud one line of three words at a time. After each line the children are asked to say which word did not begin with the target sound.

1	nine	nail	game
2	nest	hen	neck
3	dot	nose	nut
4	net	nurse	green
5	knee	ten	night
6	noon	note	snow
7	knife	pin	nip
8	newt	noise	boy
9	name	mime	nice
10	pony	nappy	nineteen
11	number	mummy	nasty
12	necklace	greasy	naughty
13	needle	ninety	dinner
14	nephew	noisy	fizzy
15	rainbow	narrow	neighbour

Odd word out — rhyming
Using a word beginning with the 'n' sound

→ The children are told to listen for the word that does not rhyme with the other two. They then listen while the teacher reads aloud one line of three words at a time. After each line the children are asked to say which word does not rhyme with the other two.

→ Alternatively, the children could be asked to say which two words do rhyme.

→ As an extra task, the children could think of other words that rhyme with the two rhyming words in each set.

1	net	fin	pet
2	nail	tail	boil
3	white	night	wine
4	nut	bat	hut
5	name	lame	team
6	pack	neck	deck
7	fast	nest	best
8	nurse	horse	purse
9	time	nine	line
10	nappy	floppy	happy

Words to sound out for the 'n' sound

→ Only words with regular spelling have been included.

→ The teacher takes one word at a time and 'sounds out' each phoneme. This may need to be done several times. The children must then guess what the word is. Some children may be able to try writing the word.

→ The children may like to repeat the phonemes consecutively, just as the teacher did, to help them blend the sounds into words.

n—e—t	n—u—t	n—ai—l	n—e—ck
n—e—s—t	n—oo—n	n—o—t	n—ee—d

Story for the 'n' sound

→ The teacher asks the children to listen carefully to the story and pick out the words beginning with the target sound. The teacher then reads the story, sentence by sentence. After each sentence the teacher asks the children:
  – To say how many words they heard beginning with the given sound in that sentence.
  – To repeat the words they heard beginning with the target sound.

→ Alternatively, the teacher can slowly read the whole story, and the children can make a tally mark on a piece of paper every time they hear a word beginning with the target sound. The children can then count up how many words they have heard beginning with that sound and tell the teacher what those words are.

The necklace

Noah was a newspaper boy. He needed some money to buy a new laptop computer. So far Noah had saved £90. Every day Noah, on his nice new bike, delivered 39 newspapers. One day, on his rounds, Noah noticed something shiny in the road and braked sharply. Unfortunately, he came off his bike, cutting his knee and grazing his knuckles and his nose. Noah knelt on the ground and saw that the shiny object was a necklace. Noah was outside some flats in Nelson Court. He got up and left his bike against a notice telling people not to walk on the grass. Noah knocked on all the doors in Nelson Court. He asked the people if they had lost a necklace. At last Noah found the owner of the necklace. It was Nicola, the nurse, who lived at flat number 19. Her nephew, Nathan, had thrown the necklace out of the window. She gave Noah nine £5 notes as a reward. Nicola also gently cleaned the cut on his knee and the grazes on his knuckles and nose.

Puzzle worksheet for the 'n' sound

Use the 'n' pictures to help you with these puzzles.

Unscramble the words below. They all begin with 'n'.

1 tnu   **2** cnke   **3** alni   **4** reusn   **5** endele

_____   _____   _____   _____   _____

Look for the 'n' words in the wordsearch below. They can read down or across. There are eight 'n' words of three letters or more.

q	r	n	v	h	w	g	n
x	d	e	m	k	n	r	o
n	y	c	p	j	e	b	s
i	f	k	w	n	e	t	e
n	a	i	l	v	d	z	b
e	s	w	r	t	l	p	o
n	u	r	s	e	e	x	g
n	e	s	t	y	j	f	l

Write down the words that you found:

1 _____   2 _____

3 _____   4 _____

5 _____   6 _____

7 _____   8 _____

Illustrations for the 'n' sound

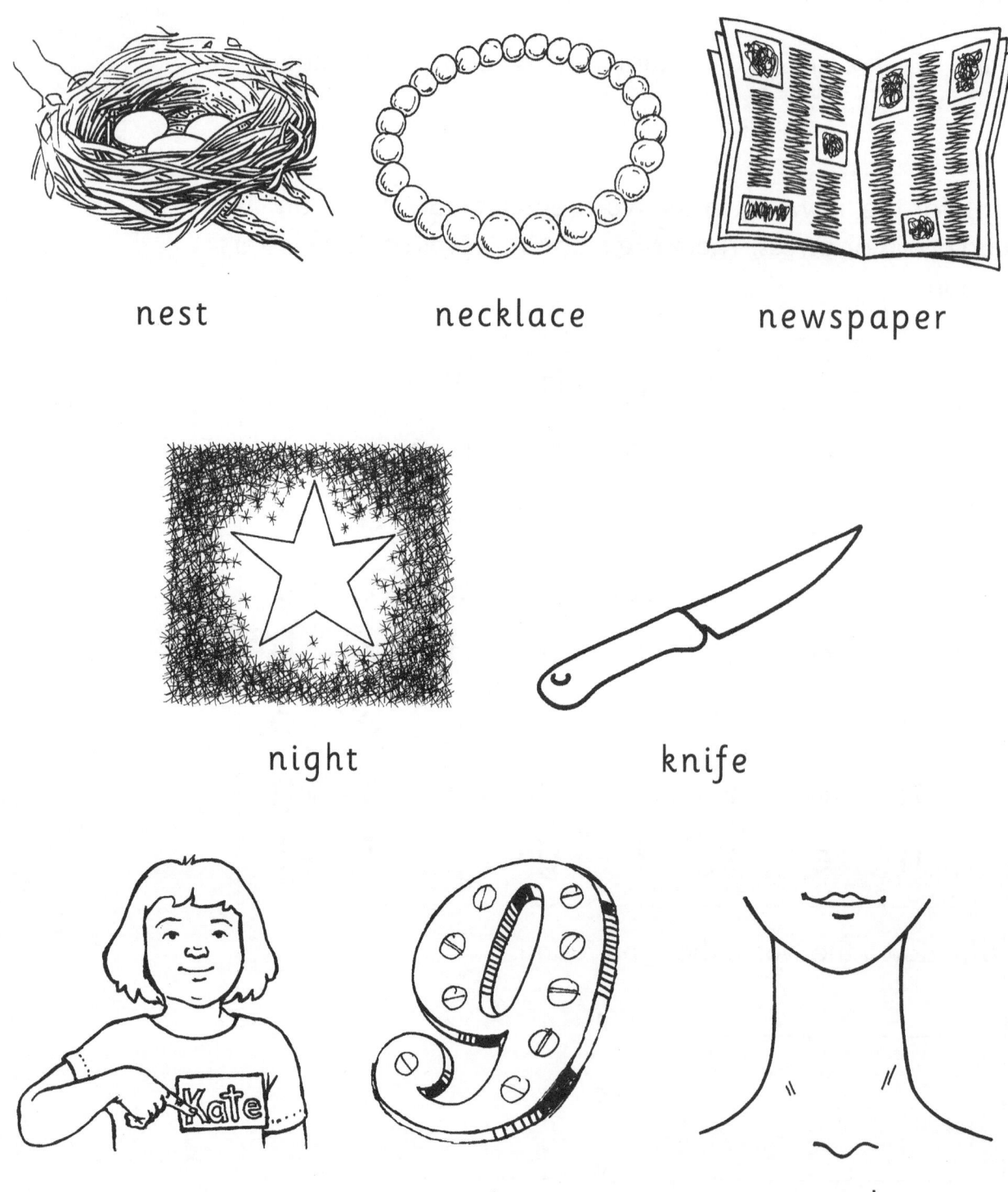

nest

necklace

newspaper

night

knife

name

nine

neck

Illustrations for the 'n' sound

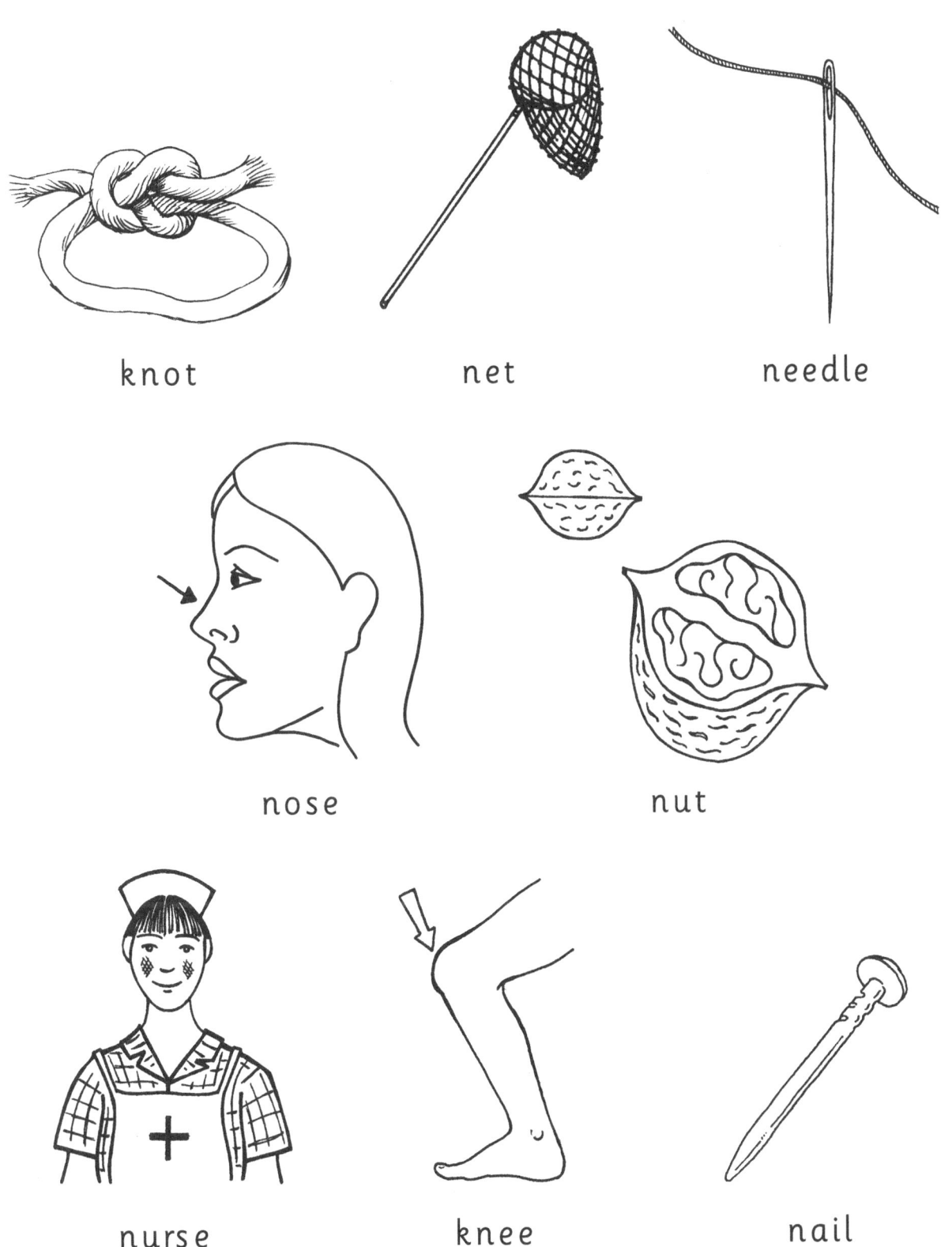

knot

net

needle

nose

nut

nurse

knee

nail

Section for the 'p' sound

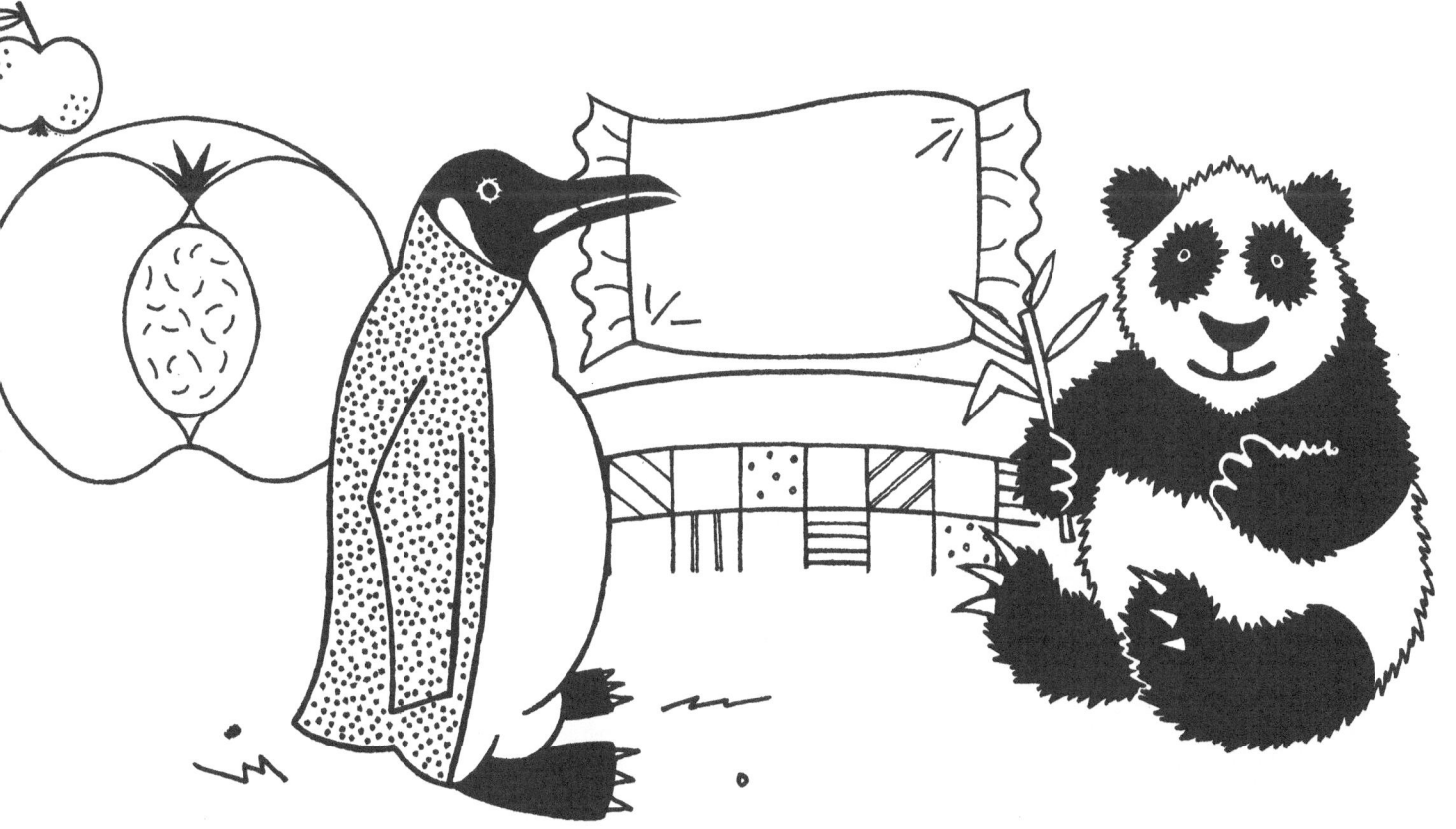

Section for the 'p' sound

Riddles for the 'p' sound

→ Children are given the photocopied pictures to go with the target sound. The teacher reads out the riddles, one at a time, and the children decide which picture each one refers to. If desired, the children can then colour these pictures in.

→ *To make the activity more difficult*, the children, without access to the pictures, are told the target sound, and the riddles are read out one at a time. The children have to think of something that starts with that sound and fits in with the riddle.

→ *To teach vocabulary*, the teacher and the children look together at the photocopied pictures, and the teacher names and talks about each illustration. The teacher then proceeds to read out the riddles as suggested above.

1   You can eat this. It is a green vegetable. (*pea*)
2   This is a bird. It lives where it is very cold. (*penguin*)
3   It is made of metal. It has a head and a point. (*pin*)
4   It is an animal. It is furry and black and white. (*panda*)
5   This is soft. You put your head on it. (*pillow*)
6   This could be lots of colours. You use a brush with it. (*paint*)
7   This is an animal. It lives in a sty. (*pig*)
8   You can eat this. It has a big stone in the middle. (*peach*)
9   This is a vegetable. You can boil, fry or roast it. (*potato*)
10   You can write with this. You can sharpen it. (*pencil*)
11   You put things in it. You might have one in your coat. (*pocket*)
12   This is a bird. It is sometimes kept in a cage. (*parrot*)

Alliteration for the 'p' sound

→ The teacher states what the target sound is. They then read out each two-word phrase, and, after each one, the children must say whether one word or both words start with the target sound.

→ Alternatively, the teacher can give each child two cards with the target sound printed on. If both words in the phrase begin with the target sound, the children hold up two cards. If only one begins with that sound, they hold up one card.

sharp pin	pink pig
purple pencil	pointed hat
painted wall	poor parrot
green peas	mashed potato
pale face	patterned pillow
patient penguin	polished piano

Tongue twisters for the 'p' sound

→ The teacher reads each tongue twister aloud and, after each one, asks the children to repeat it once or twice.

→ The children can play a game of Chinese Whispers. The teacher whispers the tongue twister to one child; this child whispers it to the next and so on. The last child says out loud what they think the teacher said, and this is compared with the original tongue twister.

1 Paige passed the purple packet of peas to Petra.
2 Polly purchased a pearl pendant in Paris.
3 The parrot pecked at the pear and pecan pie.
4 The plumber played with the plain plastic plugs.
5 The pretty princess presented the prawns to the prince.

Odd word out – initial sounds

Involving words beginning with the 'p' sound

→ The children are told which initial sound to listen for. They then listen while the teacher reads aloud one line of three words at a time. After each line the children are asked to say which word did not begin with the target sound.

1	paint	joint	pen
2	pea	pear	kite
3	door	peach	pond
4	peel	yard	park
5	pin	park	foot
6	pig	goose	pail
7	peg	pipe	sweep
8	pink	sock	pack
9	pepper	paper	ladder
10	apple	pickle	petal
11	puppy	poppy	happy
12	turnip	pocket	parrot
13	penguin	pillow	swallow
14	potato	tomato	pelican
15	pyjamas	pineapple	bananas

Odd word out — rhyming
Using a word beginning with the 'p' sound

→ The children are told to listen for the word that does not rhyme with the other two. They then listen while the teacher reads aloud one line of three words at a time. After each line the children are asked to say which word does not rhyme with the other two.

→ Alternatively, the children could be asked to say which two words do rhyme.

→ As an extra task, the children could think of other words that rhyme with the two rhyming words in each set.

1	fin	bee	pea
2	hen	sit	pen
3	pig	bag	wig
4	wait	plate	rain
5	pet	cat	wet
6	heel	pear	wear
7	pin	man	win
8	peach	beach	patch
9	racket	pocket	rocket
10	parrot	carrot	ferret

Words to sound out for the 'p' sound

→ Only words with regular spelling have been included.

→ The teacher takes one word at a time and 'sounds out' each phoneme. This may need to be done several times. The children must then guess what the word is. Some children may be able to try writing the word.

→ The children may like to repeat the phonemes consecutively, just as the teacher did, to help them blend the sounds into words.

p—ea	p—e—n	p—i—n	p—ea—ch
p—i—g	p—o—n—d	p—ai—n—t	p—ar—k

Story for the 'p' sound

→ The teacher asks the children to listen carefully to the story and pick out the words beginning with the target sound. The teacher then reads the story, sentence by sentence. After each sentence the teacher asks the children:
  – To say how many words they heard beginning with the given sound in that sentence.
  – To repeat the words they heard beginning with the target sound.
→ Alternatively, the teacher can slowly read the whole story, and the children can make a tally mark on a piece of paper every time they hear a word beginning with the target sound. The children can then count up how many words they have heard beginning with that sound and tell the teacher what those words are.

The wet paint

Pedro's mum asked him to go to the post office to purchase a stamp.

To get to the post office Pedro walked through a passage to a park.

On the way through the park Pedro passed lots of people. He passed

a boy riding a pony, a lady wearing a pale blue coat and a little girl

with a pet parrot on her arm. The parrot was pecking at the girl's

pocket. Pedro paused for a moment and perched on a park bench. He

did not see the notice that said 'WET PAINT'. Pedro stayed there

watching the people playing cricket on the grass by the pond. When

Pedro stood up, his purple jumper had pink stripes on the back of it.

He proceeded to the post office and purchased a stamp. Pedro went

back home via the park and the passage. Pedro's mother was

pleased that he had purchased the stamp but was not pleased

when she saw the pink stripes on his purple jumper.

Puzzle worksheet for the 'p' sound

Use the 'p' pictures to help you with these puzzles.

Unscramble the words below. They all begin with 'p'.

1 pne   **2** gpi   **3** eapr   **4** aadpn   **5** pppeer

_____   _____   _____   _____   _____

Look for the 'p' words in the wordsearch below. They can read down or across. There are eight 'p' words of three letters or more.

w	p	r	t	y	u	z	p
k	i	p	o	n	d	r	a
j	g	h	g	f	d	p	n
z	p	a	i	n	t	a	d
o	q	s	d	c	x	r	a
n	p	n	p	e	a	r	m
y	e	w	f	s	k	o	z
c	n	x	p	l	a	t	e

Write down the words that you found:

1 _____   2 _____

3 _____   4 _____

5 _____   6 _____

7 _____   8 _____

Illustrations for the 'p' sound

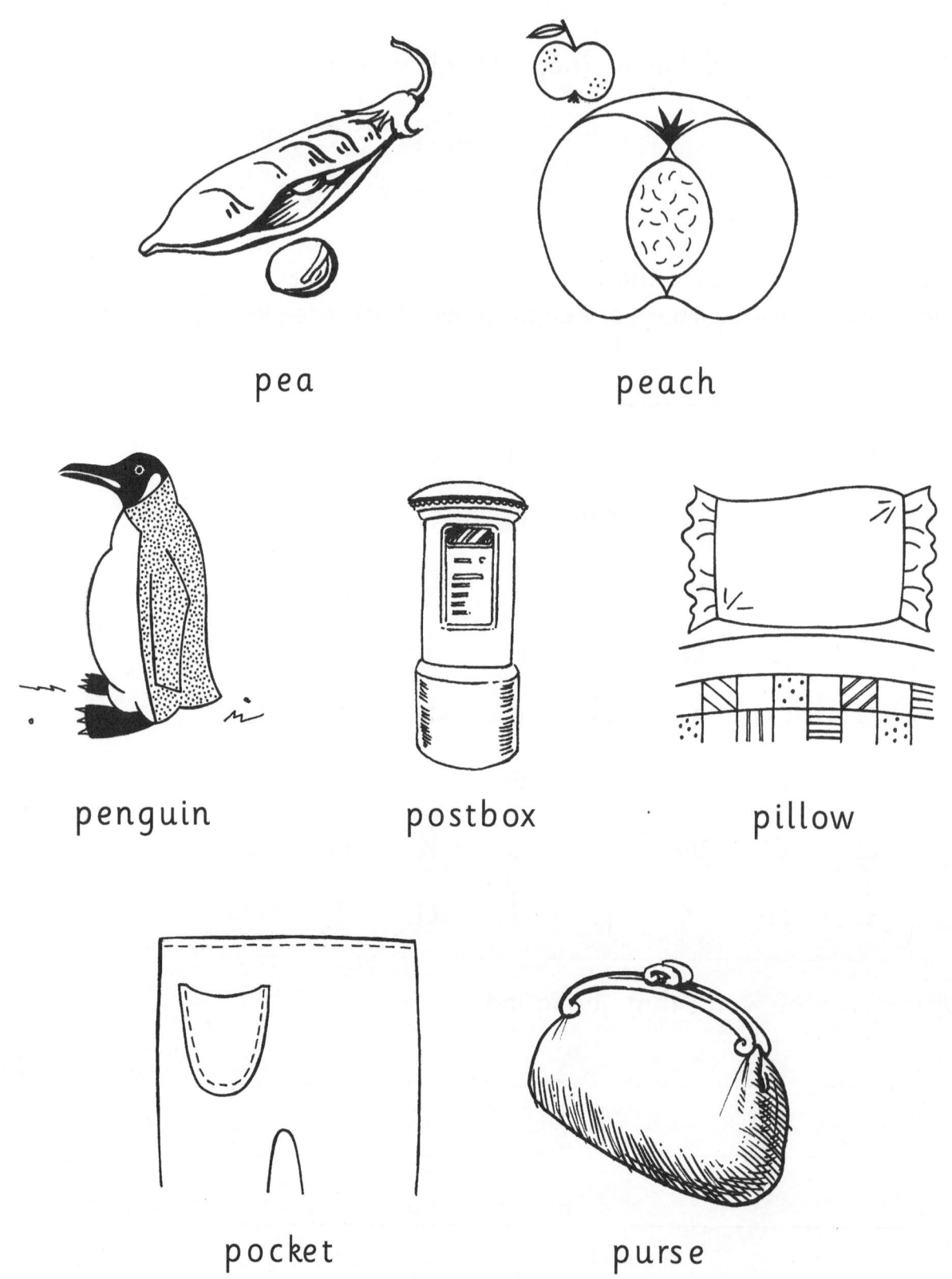

pea

peach

penguin

postbox

pillow

pocket

purse

Illustrations for the 'p' sound

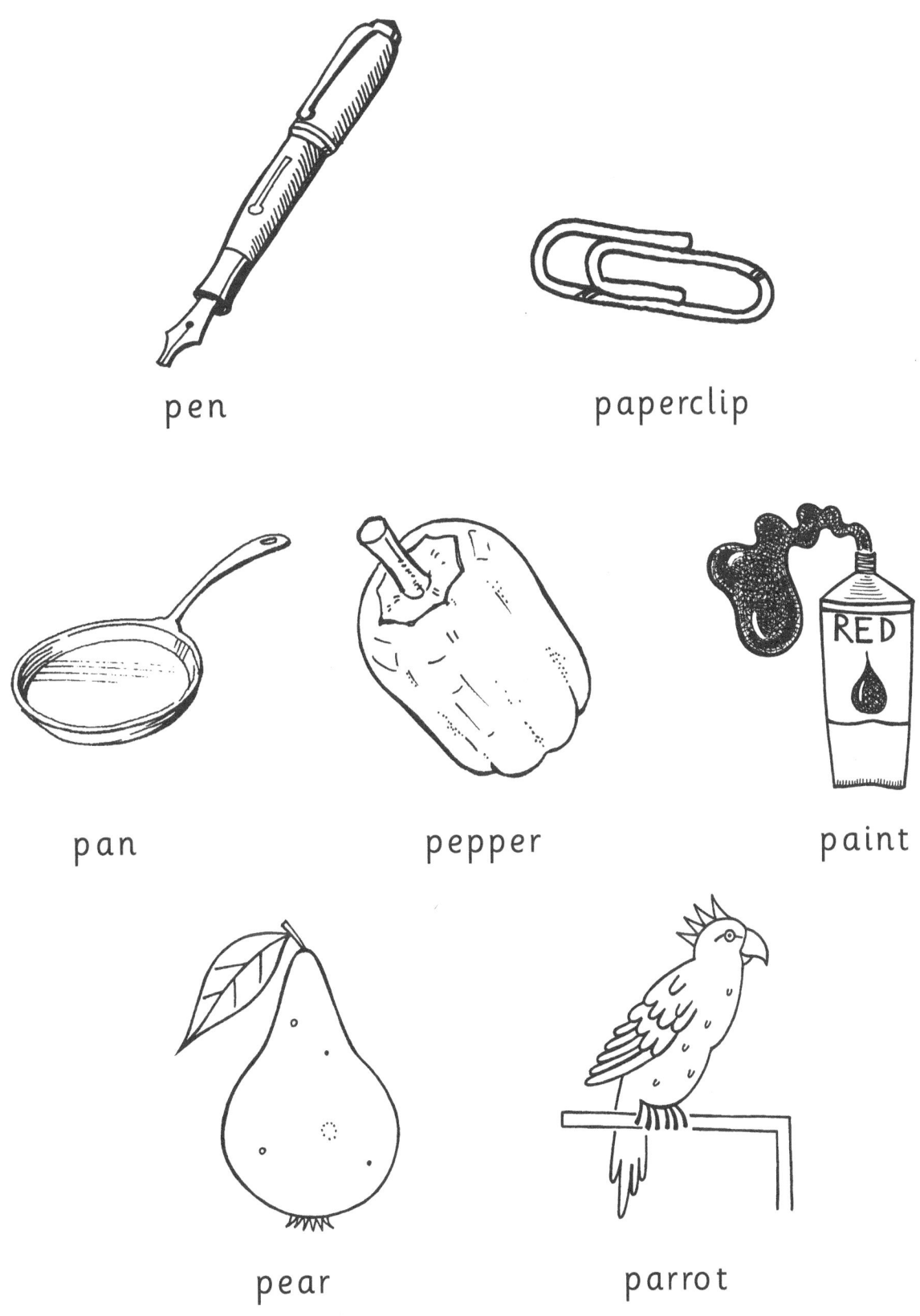

pen

paperclip

pan

pepper

RED

paint

pear

parrot

2/3

Illustrations for the 'p' sound

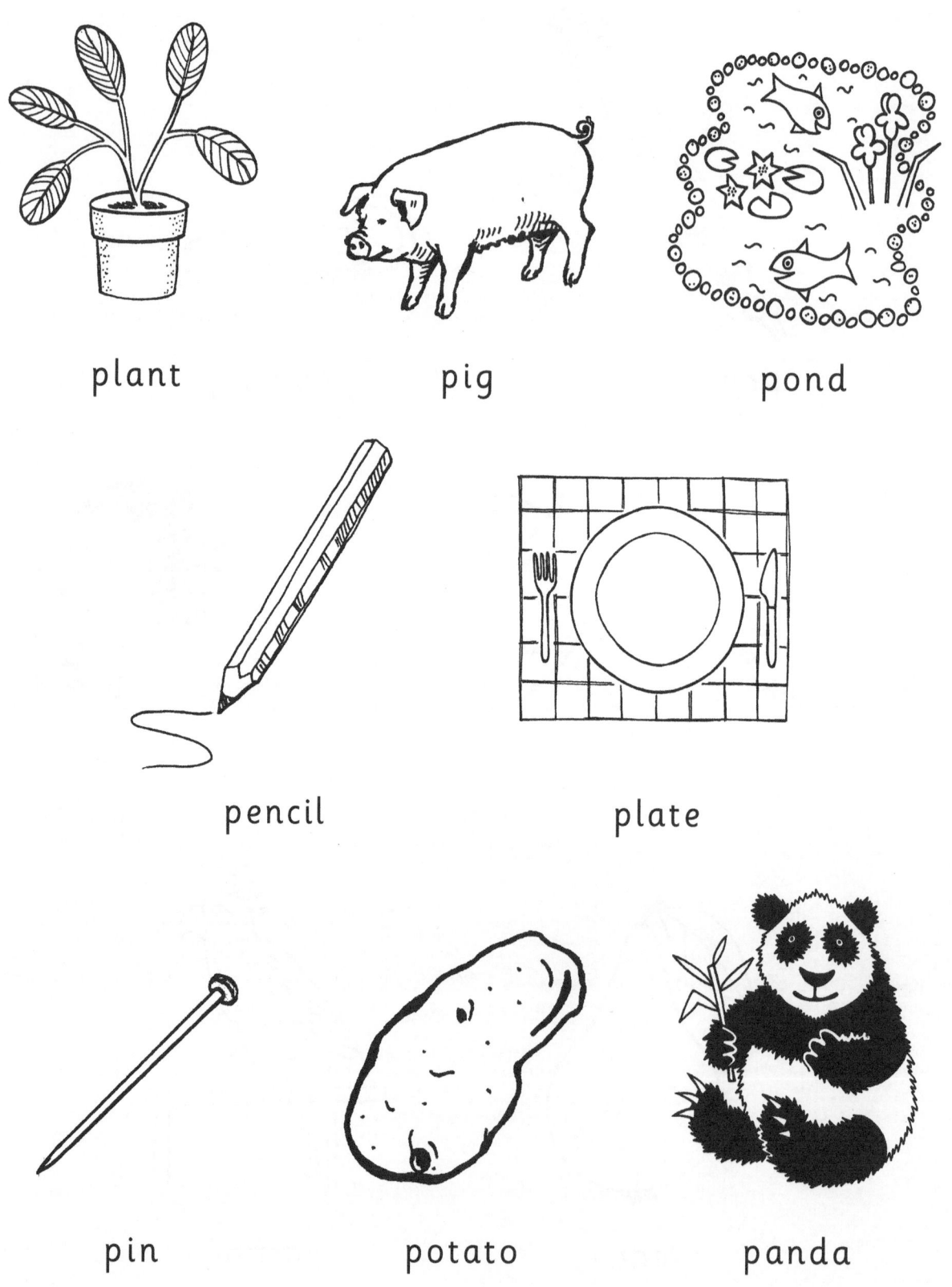

plant

pig

pond

pencil

plate

pin

potato

panda

Section for the 'r' sound

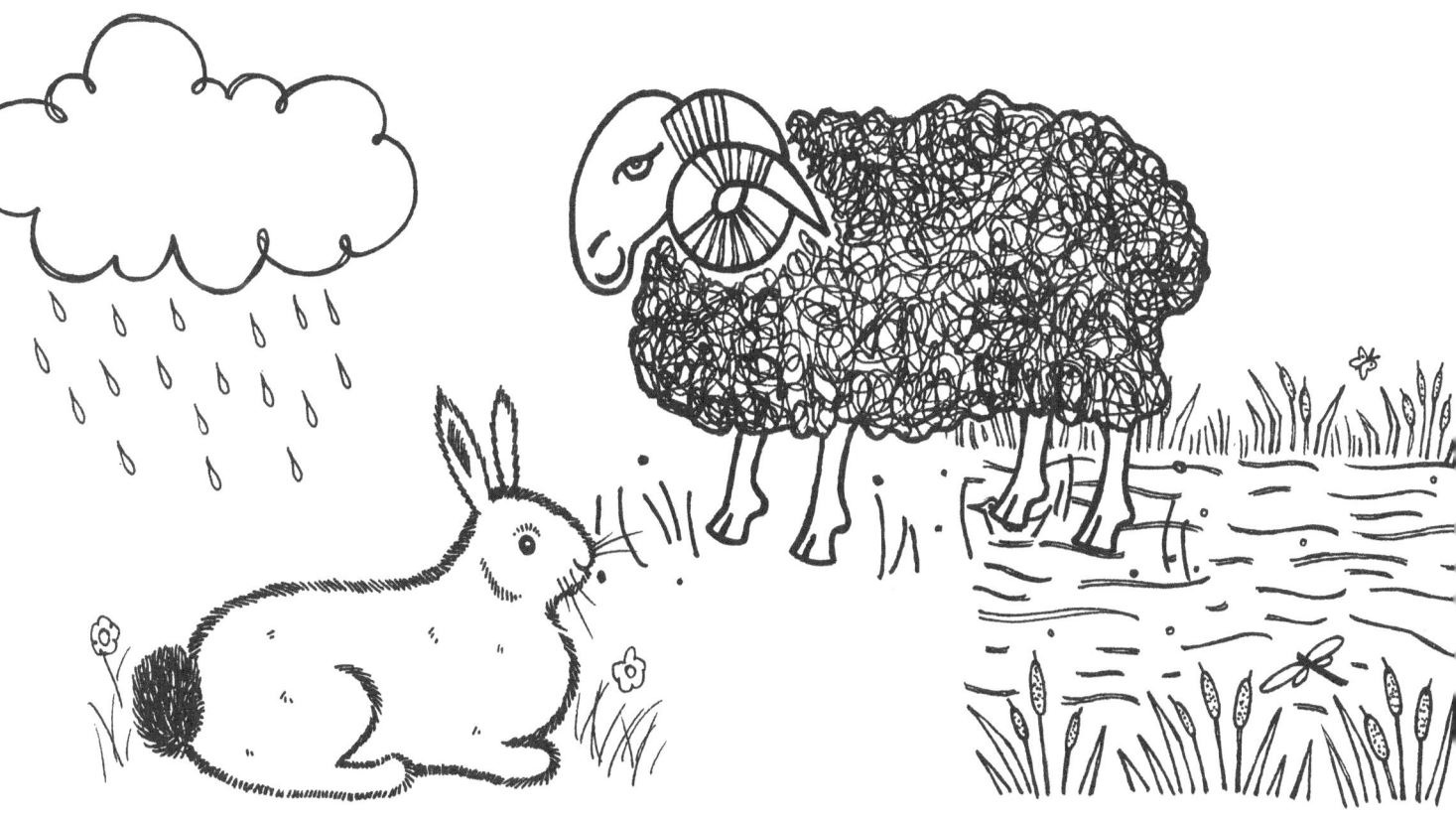

Section for the 'r' sound

Suitable for children in Year R

Riddles for the 'r' sound

→ Children are given the photocopied pictures to go with the target sound. The teacher reads out the riddles, one at a time, and the children decide which picture each one refers to. If desired, the children can then colour these pictures in.

→ *To make the activity more difficult*, the children, without access to the pictures, are told the target sound, and the riddles are read out one at a time. The children have to think of something that starts with that sound and fits in with the riddle.

→ *To teach vocabulary*, the teacher and the children look together at the photocopied pictures, and the teacher names and talks about each illustration. The teacher then proceeds to read out the riddles as suggested above.

1   This is an animal. It has a woolly coat and sometimes it has horns. (*ram*)
2   This is a tool. You might use it in the garden. (*rake*)
3   This has water in it. It might have fish in it or a boat on it. (*river*)
4   This is long. You might use it to tie a boat up with. (*rope*)
5   You can turn this on or off. You can hear music or voices coming from it. (*radio*)
6   This has two legs. Sometimes it has a red breast. (*robin*)
7   You can eat this. It might have a filling in the middle. (*roll*)
8   It goes up into space. It makes a lot of noise. (*rocket*)
9   This comes from the sky. It makes things wet. (*rain*)
10   You have to look up to see this. It is part of a house. (*roof*)
11   It has four sides. It has four corners. (*rectangle*)
12   This is an animal. It has long ears and likes to eat carrots and lettuce. (*rabbit*)

Alliteration for the 'r' sound

Suitable for children in Years R, 1 and 2

→ The teacher states what the target sound is. They then read out each two-word phrase, and, after each one, the children must say whether one word or both words start with the target sound.

→ Alternatively, the teacher can give each child two cards with the target sound printed on. If both words in the phrase begin with the target sound, the children hold up two cards. If only one begins with that sound, they hold up one card.

fried rice	raw meat
red rose	real rabbit
rich lady	right hand
rude boy	rough road
round rug	rainy day
pretty rainbow	ruby ring

Tongue twisters for the 'r' sound

Suitable for children in Years R, 1 and 2

→ The teacher reads each tongue twister aloud and, after each one, asks the children to repeat it once or twice.

→ The children can play a game of Chinese Whispers. The teacher whispers the tongue twister to one child; this child whispers it to the next and so on. The last child says out loud what they think the teacher said, and this is compared with the original tongue twister.

1 The rain rolled down Ryan's red raincoat.
2 Regan received a ruby ring in a red rose.
3 Ruben rowed to the rocks and rescued the rabbit.
4 The robot rotated and raced to the rusty rocket.
5 Robbie rushed to retrieve the red rake.

Odd word out – initial sounds

Involving words beginning with the 'r' sound

→ The children are told which initial sound to listen for. They then listen while the teacher reads aloud one line of three words at a time. After each line the children are asked to say which word did not begin with the target sound.

1	rice	rain	two
2	rake	hut	rat
3	road	dig	rug
4	root	ram	watch
5	yacht	rock	roof
6	red	leg	rag
7	run	pond	rock
8	rose	roll	owl
9	bike	right	race
10	ribbon	letter	rocket
11	rainbow	rabbit	adder
12	ruler	tractor	ruby
13	rusty	radio	dragon
14	robot	rattle	butter
15	river	diver	robin

Odd word out — rhyming
Using a word beginning with the 'r' sound

➜ The children are told to listen for the word that does not rhyme with the other two. They then listen while the teacher reads aloud one line of three words at a time. After each line the children are asked to say which word does not rhyme with the other two.

➜ Alternatively, the children could be asked to say which two words do rhyme.

➜ As an extra task, the children could think of other words that rhyme with the two rhyming words in each set.

1	ring	lane	wing
2	mug	rake	cake
3	rock	clock	ham
4	rose	peas	nose
5	cloud	road	toad
6	rang	sang	swing
7	fought	right	night
8	ham	comb	ram
9	ten	ran	pan
10	rain	coin	lane

Words to sound out for the 'r' sound

➜ Only words with regular spelling have been included.

➜ The teacher takes one word at a time and 'sounds out' each phoneme. This may need to be done several times. The children must then guess what the word is. Some children may be able to try writing the word.

➜ The children may like to repeat the phonemes consecutively, just as the teacher did, to help them blend the sounds into words.

r—a—t	r—u—g	r—a—m	r—oo—t
r—o—ck	r—oo—f	r—oa—d	r—u—n

Story for the 'r' sound

→ The teacher asks the children to listen carefully to the story and pick out the words beginning with the target sound. The teacher then reads the story, sentence by sentence. After each sentence the teacher asks the children:

- To say how many words they heard beginning with the given sound in that sentence.
- To repeat the words they heard beginning with the target sound.

→ Alternatively, the teacher can slowly read the whole story, and the children can make a tally mark on a piece of paper every time they hear a word beginning with the target sound. The children can then count up how many words they have heard beginning with that sound and tell the teacher what those words are.

Ruby's ring

Ruby was walking along the road by the river in the rain. Some horrible black rats ran across the road in front of Ruby. Ruby was startled, and she started to run. It was raining very fast, so Ruby took off her gloves to pull up the hood of her raincoat. As she did this her red ring came off her finger, and she thought it must have rolled down the river bank. Ruby was upset, but she remembered that her friend Ria had a metal detector. She ran to Ria's house in Regent Road and rang the doorbell. Ria opened the door, and Ruby told her about the ring. Together Ruby and Ria set off for the river bank. Ria swept the metal detector over the reeds and grass. The metal detector found a metal object and made a ringing noise. Ria rested the detector against a rock. Both girls ran their hands through the rough reeds. They found lots of rubbish but no ring. Ria and Ruby gave up looking for the ring and returned home. On reaching her house, Ruby went inside and took off her raincoat. As she did so, her red ring fell out of the sleeve of her raincoat.

Puzzle worksheet for the 'r' sound

Use the 'r' pictures to help you with these puzzles.

Unscramble the words below. They all begin with 'r'.

1 mra   **2** arni   **3** peor   **4** rrvie   **5** ctekro

_____   _____   _____   _____   _____

Look for the 'r' words in the wordsearch below. They can read down or across. There are eight 'r' words of three or more letters.

r	a	b	b	i	t	w	r
i	z	e	r	s	x	r	o
b	d	c	a	t	f	v	c
b	y	r	i	n	g	h	k
o	u	b	n	i	j	n	e
n	p	k	b	m	r	a	t
l	w	r	o	a	d	g	v
x	j	y	w	q	r	u	g

Write down the words that you found:

1 _____   2 _____

3 _____   4 _____

5 _____   6 _____

7 _____   8 _____

123

Illustrations for the 'r' sound

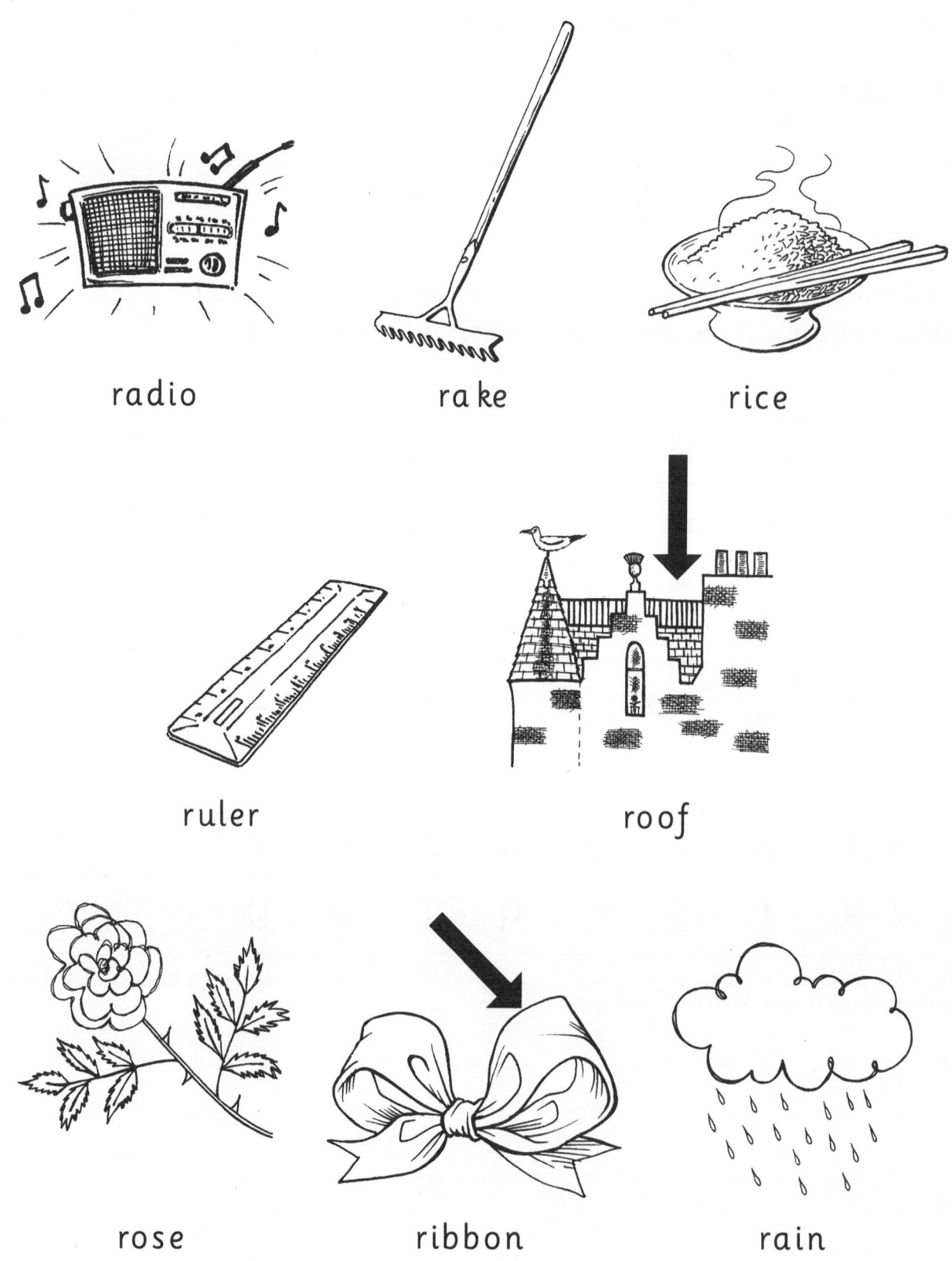

radio

rake

rice

ruler

roof

rose

ribbon

rain

Illustrations for the 'r' sound

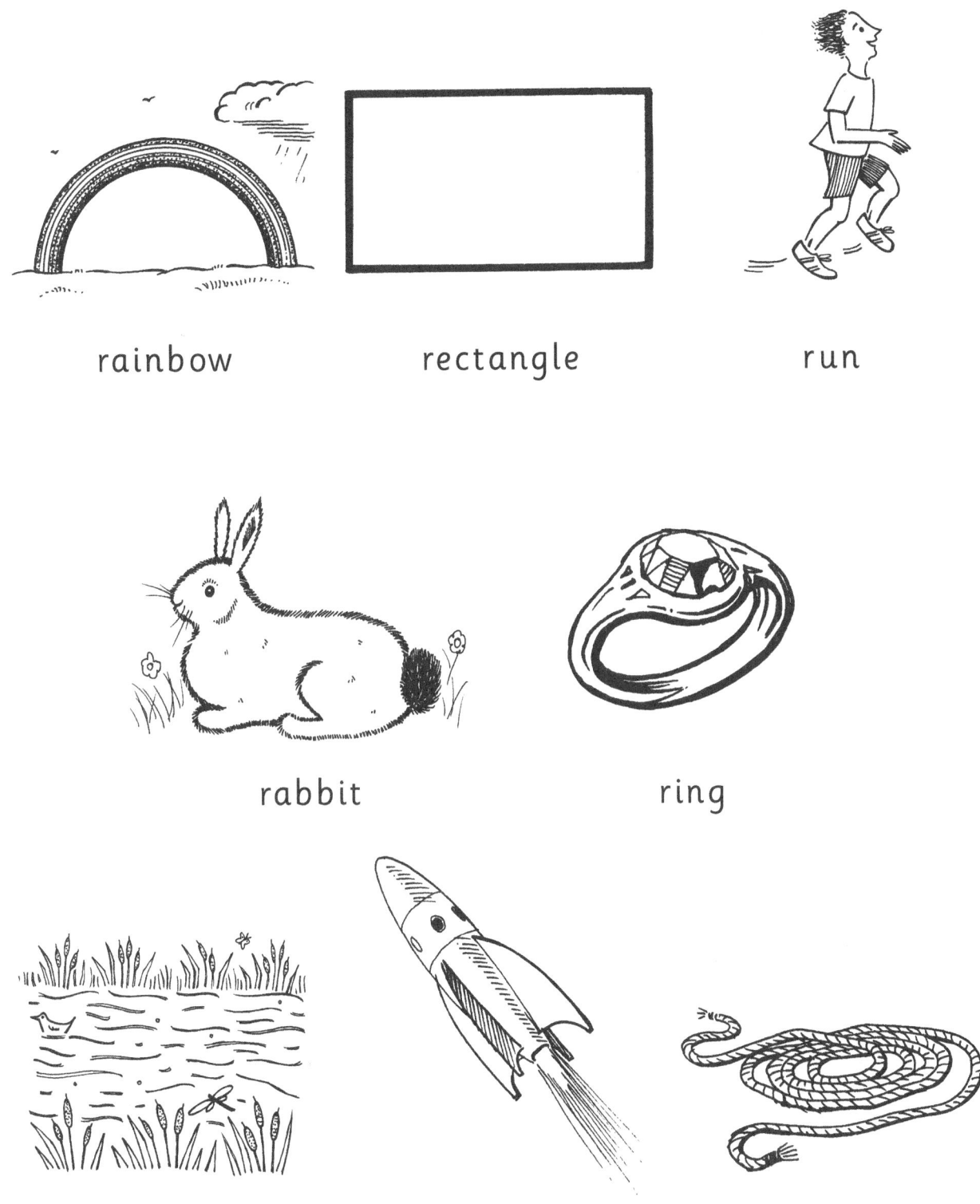

rainbow

rectangle

run

rabbit

ring

river

rocket

rope

Illustrations for the 'r' sound

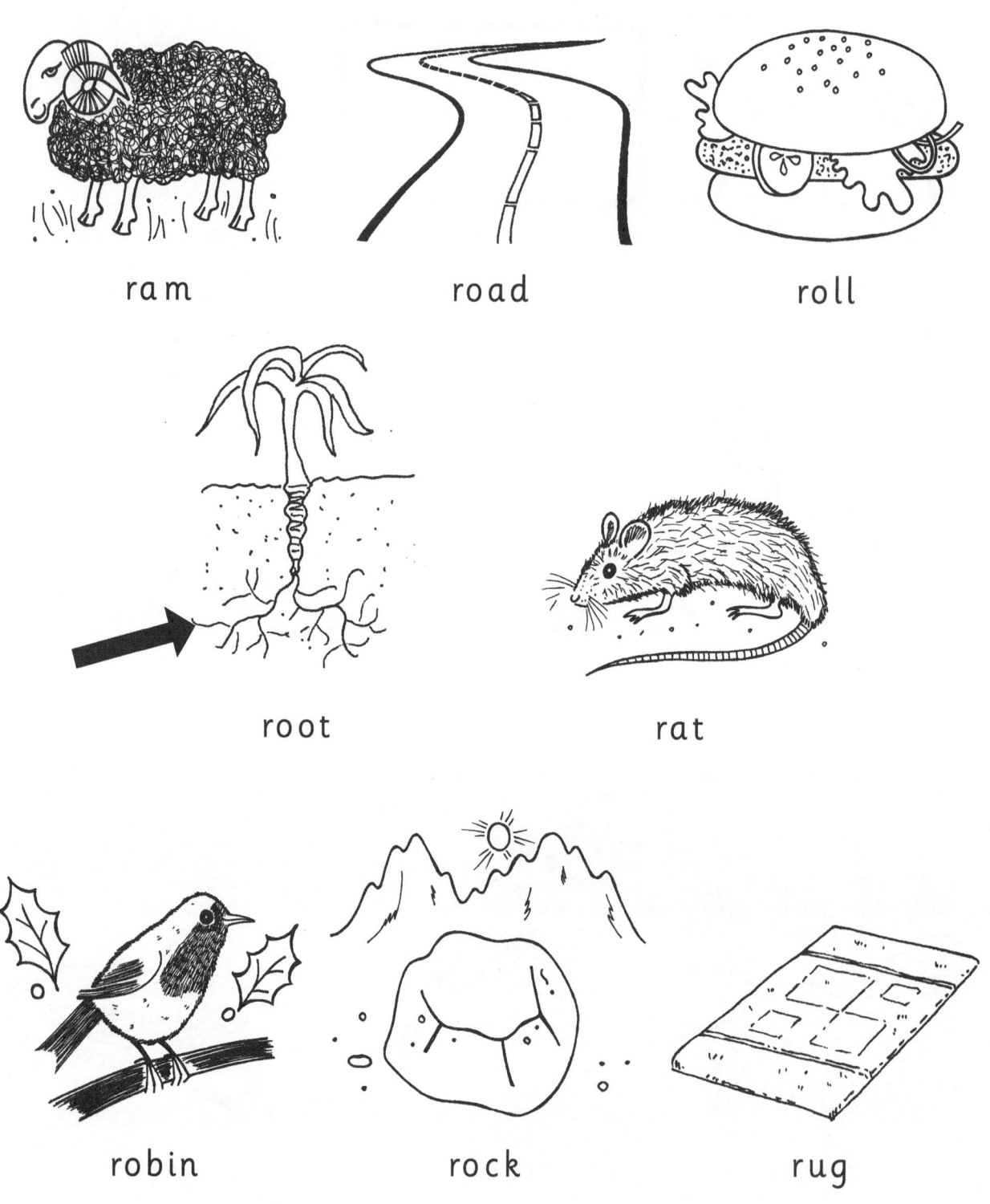

ram

road

roll

root

rat

robin

rock

rug

Section for the 's' sound

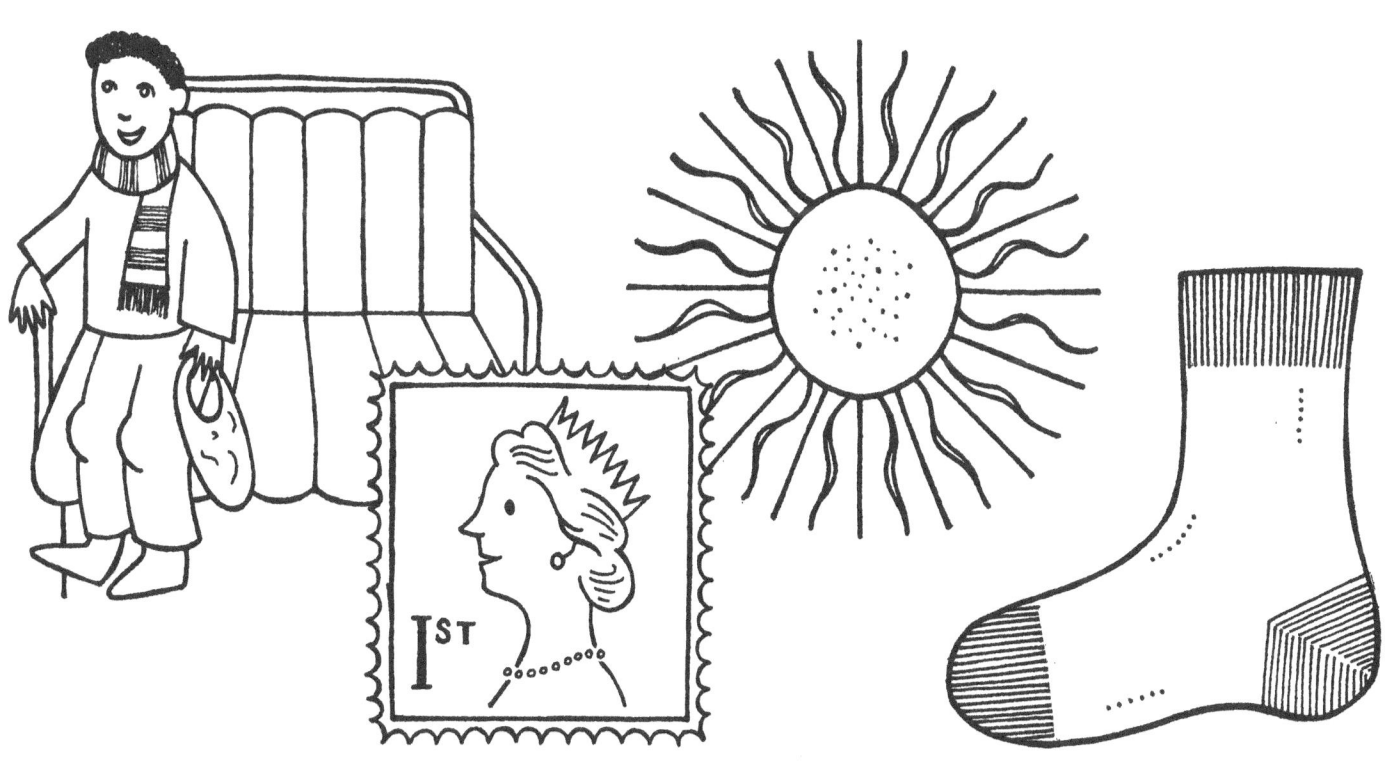

Section for the 's' sound

Riddles for the 's' sound

→ Children are given the photocopied pictures to go with the target sound. The teacher reads out the riddles, one at a time, and the children decide which picture each one refers to. If desired, the children can then colour these pictures in.

→ *To make the activity more difficult*, the children, without access to the pictures, are told the target sound, and the riddles are read out one at a time. The children have to think of something that starts with that sound and fits in with the riddle.

→ *To teach vocabulary*, the teacher and the children look together at the photocopied pictures, and the teacher names and talks about each illustration. The teacher then proceeds to read out the riddles as suggested above.

1 This is a number. An insect has this many legs. (*six*)
2 This can swim in the sea. It likes eating fish. (*seal*)
3 You sit on this when you ride a horse. A bicycle also has one. (*saddle*)
4 This is a number. There are this many days in a week. (*seven*)
5 This has lots of teeth. You use this for cutting wood. (*saw*)
6 This might be hot. You eat it with a spoon. (*soup*)
7 This can be pulled up or down. A yacht has one. (*sail*)
8 This has a plug hole. It also has one or two taps. (*sink*)
9 This is white. You sprinkle it on food. (*salt*)
10 You can eat these. They are made from meat. (*sausages*)
11 These are made of metal. They can be very sharp. (*scissors*)
12 You might paddle in it. Seals and other creatures swim in it. (*sea*)

Alliteration for the 's' sound

Suitable for children in Years R, 1 and 2

→ The teacher states what the target sound is. They then read out each two-word phrase, and, after each one, the children must say whether one word or both words start with the target sound.

→ Alternatively, the teacher can give each child two cards with the target sound printed on. If both words in the phrase begin with the target sound, the children hold up two cards. If only one begins with that sound, they hold up one card.

sad seal	tinned soup
hot sun	six socks
silly sailor	soapy water
muddy sole	silver sword
seven saucers	wooden seat
salty sausages	soft soap

Tongue twisters for the 's' sound

Suitable for children in Years R, 1 and 2

→ The teacher reads each tongue twister aloud and, after each one, asks the children to repeat it once or twice.

→ The children can play a game of Chinese Whispers. The teacher whispers the tongue twister to one child; this child whispers it to the next and so on. The last child says out loud what they think the teacher said, and this is compared with the original tongue twister.

1 The sailor saved seven sad sick seals.
2 The skier skidded into the skinny scarecrow.
3 The slimy slug slept in my slippers.
4 The snoring snake snoozed in the snow.
5 The spotty spaniel spied the spinning spider.

Odd word out — initial sounds

Involving words beginning with the 's' sound

→ The children are told which initial sound to listen for. They then listen while the teacher reads aloud one line of three words at a time. After each line the children are asked to say which word did not begin with the target sound.

1	sack	sand	ring
2	seal	thorn	saw
3	sat	goose	sole
4	sink	soup	shirt
5	coat	soap	salt
6	sun	seat	note
7	sail	dress	six
8	four	sea	seven
9	sauce	seed	board
10	two	sit	sew
11	sole	goat	suit
12	saddle	tiger	saucer
13	custard	sausage	sixteen
14	silver	soldier	dollar
15	scissors	pandas	sandals

Odd word out – rhyming
Using a word beginning with the 's' sound

➜ The children are told to listen for the word that does not rhyme with the other two. They then listen while the teacher reads aloud one line of three words at a time. After each line the children are asked to say which word does not rhyme with the other two.

➜ Alternatively, the children could be asked to say which two words do rhyme.

➜ As an extra task, the children could think of other words that rhyme with the two rhyming words in each set.

1	saw	tea	door
2	back	sink	pink
3	her	four	saw
4	sun	thin	bun
5	suck	truck	rock
6	food	seed	weed
7	good	suit	fruit
8	sandals	bundles	candles
9	saddle	paddle	metal
10	lemon	seven	heaven

Words to sound out for the 's' sound

➜ Only words with regular spelling have been included.

➜ The teacher takes one word at a time and 'sounds out' each phoneme. This may need to be done several times. The children must then guess what the word is. Some children may be able to try writing the word.

➜ The children may like to repeat the phonemes consecutively, just as the teacher did, to help them blend the sounds into words.

s—u—n	s—o—ck	s—oa—p	s—a—ck
s—ea—t	s—ea—l	s—a—n—d	s—ai—l

Story for the 's' sound

→ The teacher asks the children to listen carefully to the story and pick out the words beginning with the target sound. The teacher then reads the story, sentence by sentence. After each sentence the teacher asks the children:

- To say how many words they heard beginning with the given sound in that sentence.
- To repeat the words they heard beginning with the target sound.

→ Alternatively, the teacher can slowly read the whole story, and the children can make a tally mark on a piece of paper every time they hear a word beginning with the target sound. The children can then count up how many words they have heard beginning with that sound and tell the teacher what those words are.

The surfer

It was a lovely summer's day, and the sun was shining. Sydney and her sister Sophie decided to go for a picnic by the sea. So Sydney and Sophie, wearing sun hats and swimsuits, walked to the beach and sat down on the sand. Sydney made a sandcastle while Sophie put a rug on the sand and laid out the food. There were sausages, salmon sandwiches, and salt and vinegar crisps. To follow there were strawberry muffins and six sweet biscuits. After they had finished eating, Sydney and Sophie took off their sandals and went for a paddle in the sea. The two sisters stood in the water and stared out to sea. In the distance they saw a boy on a surfboard. Suddenly there was a huge wave, and the surfboarder was swept off the surfboard. The surfboarder seemed to be struggling to swim ashore. Sydney and her sister ran to a nearby life guard. They said that there was a surfboarder in trouble. The life guard, carrying a life belt, swam out to the surfboarder and saved him. When the surfboarder recovered, he thanked the two sisters for being so observant and having the sense to alert the life guard.

Puzzle worksheet for the 's' sound

Use the 's' pictures to help you with these puzzles.

Unscramble the words below. They all begin with 's'.

1 xsi   **2** lats   **3** nski   **4** upos   **5** ssgeuaa

_____   _____   _____   _____   _____

Look for the 's' words in the wordsearch below. They can read down or across. There are eight 's' words of three or more letters.

p	s	a	d	d	l	e	w
e	r	t	y	s	o	c	k
u	p	s	k	n	l	h	j
s	c	i	s	s	o	r	s
i	k	x	g	o	f	d	e
n	a	z	c	a	v	b	v
k	x	m	w	p	z	j	e
v	s	a	l	t	m	c	n

Write down the words that you found:

1 _____   2 _____

3 _____   4 _____

5 _____   6 _____

7 _____   8 _____

Illustrations for the 's' sound

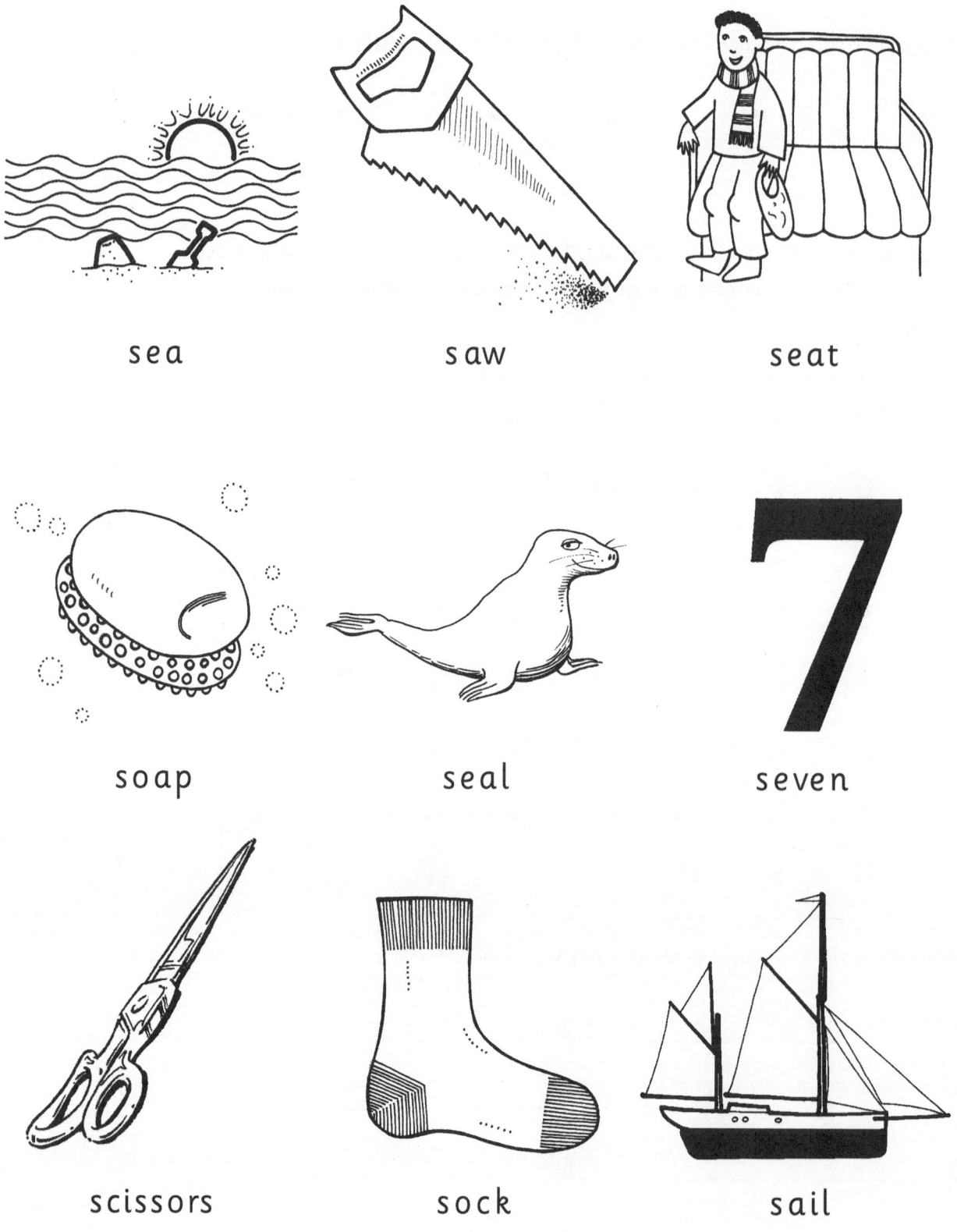

sea

saw

seat

soap

seal

seven

scissors

sock

sail

Illustrations for the 's' sound

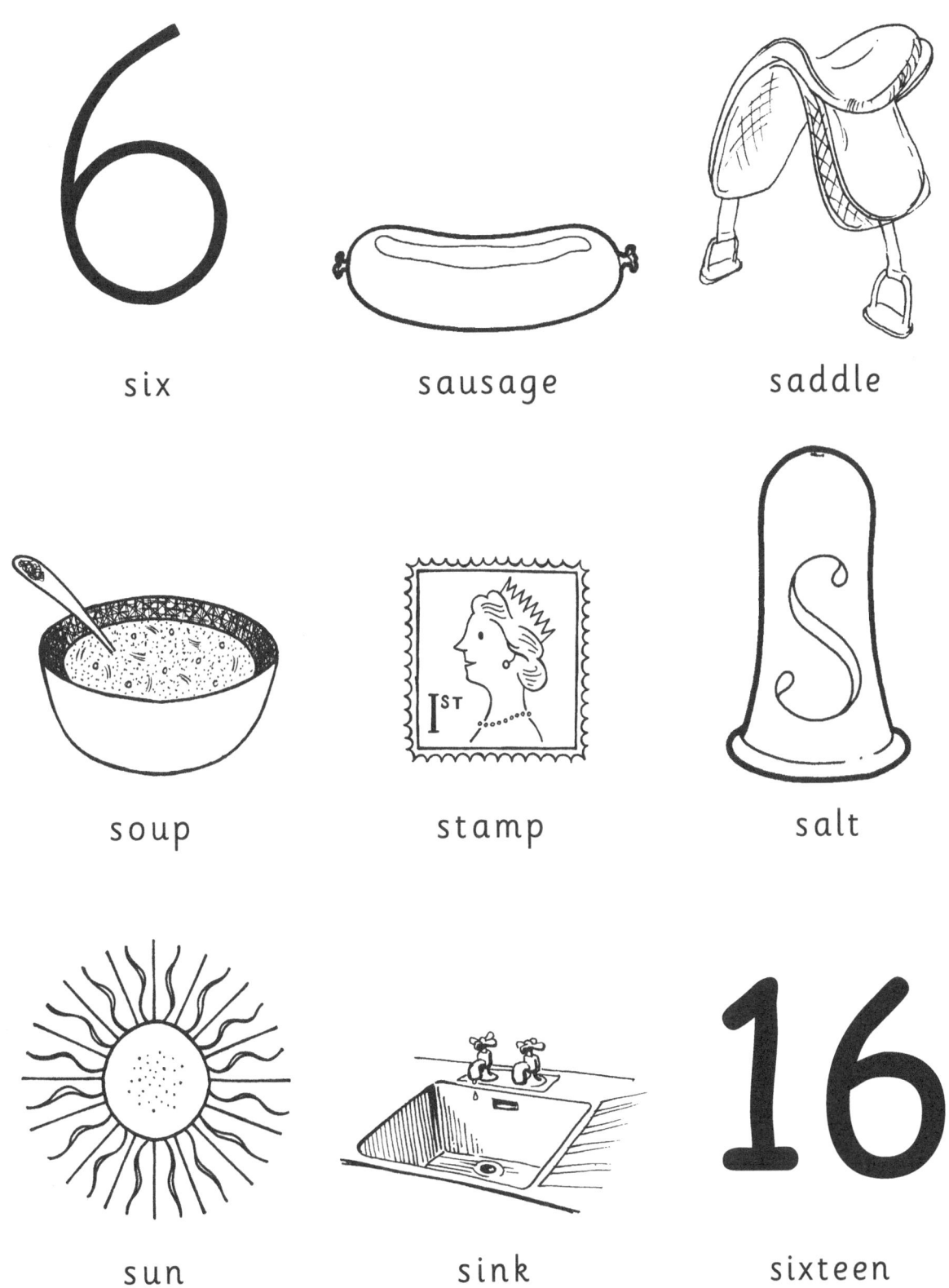

six

sausage

saddle

soup

stamp

salt

sun

sink

sixteen

2/2

Section for the 't' sound

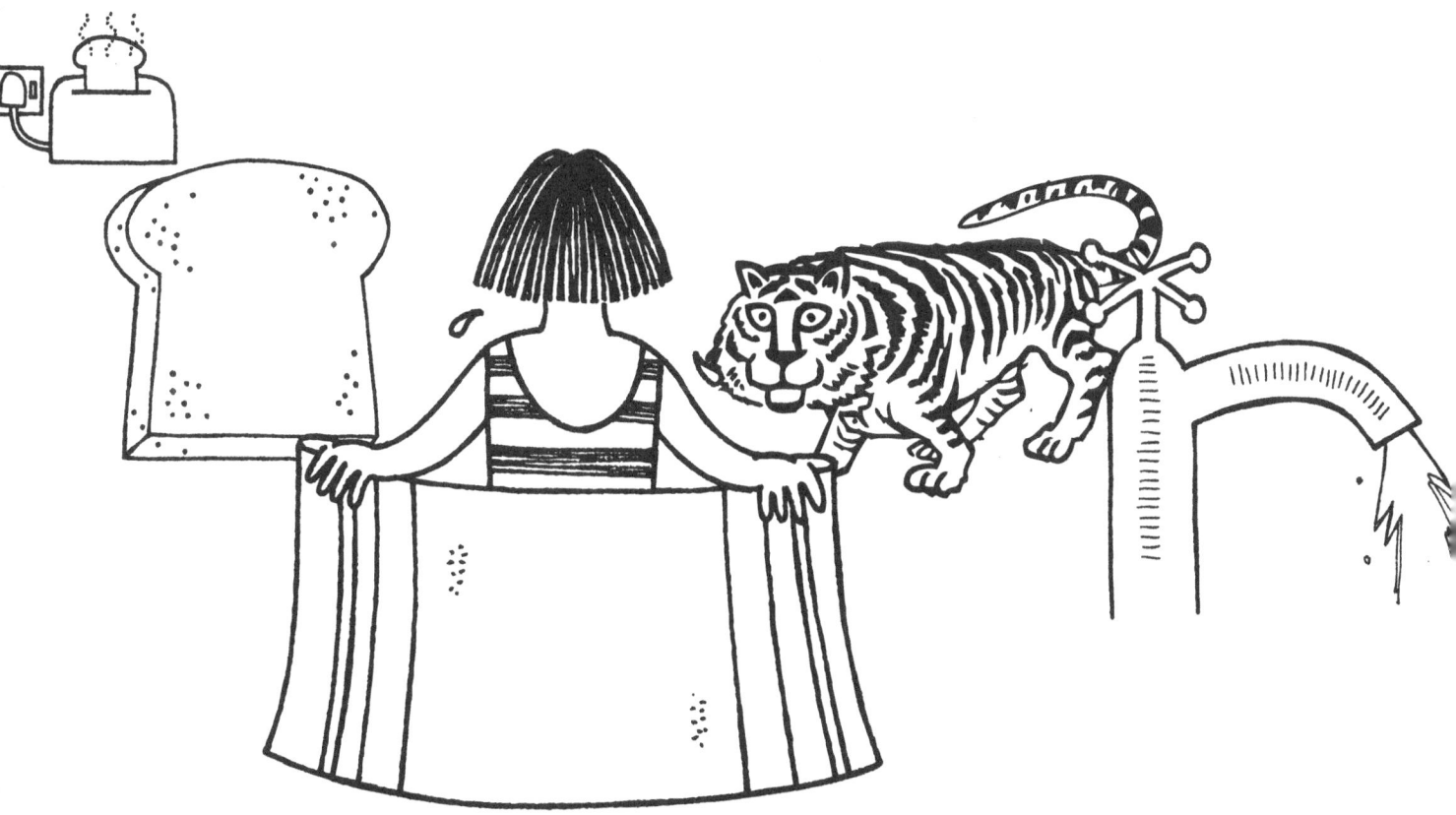

Section for the 't' sound

Riddles for the 't' sound

→ Children are given the photocopied pictures to go with the target sound. The teacher reads out the riddles, one at a time, and the children decide which picture each one refers to. If desired, the children can then colour these pictures in.

→ *To make the activity more difficult*, the children, without access to the pictures, are told the target sound, and the riddles are read out one at a time. The children have to think of something that starts with that sound and fits in with the riddle.

→ *To teach vocabulary*, the teacher and the children look together at the photocopied pictures, and the teacher names and talks about each illustration. The teacher then proceeds to read out the riddles as suggested above.

1 This has four legs. It has a top on it. (*table*)
2 You can eat this. It is red and has pips inside it. (*tomato*)
3 This is a number. You have this many toes on your feet. (*ten*)
4 This has stripes. It is fierce. (*tiger*)
5 These are like long teeth. Some animals have them. (*tusks*)
6 You might put butter on this. You might put marmalade on this. (*toast*)
7 This is a number. A turkey has this number of legs. (*two*)
8 Monkeys have one. You do not have one. (*tail*)
9 These are part of your body. You have ten of them. (*toes*)
10 Sometimes a shoe has one. You have one. (*tongue*)
11 This has a screen. You can watch it. (*television*)
12 It might be hot or cold. It might drip. (*tap*)

Alliteration for the 't' sound

→ The teacher states what the target sound is. They then read out each two-word phrase, and, after each one, the children must say whether one word or both words start with the target sound.

→ Alternatively, the teacher can give each child two cards with the target sound printed on. If both words in the phrase begin with the target sound, the children hold up two cards. If only one begins with that sound, they hold up one card.

two ties	ten cups
terrible tiger	hot tea
tall table	tired dog
tidy drawer	tiny teeth
dirty toes	tame turkey
torn towel	tomato sauce

Tongue twisters for the 't' sound

→ The teacher reads each tongue twister aloud and, after each one, asks the children to repeat it once or twice.

→ The children can play a game of Chinese Whispers. The teacher whispers the tongue twister to one child; this child whispers it to the next and so on. The last child says out loud what they think the teacher said, and this is compared with the original tongue twister.

1 Taylor took the toy tanker to Thomas.
2 Tony tiptoed timidly to the television.
3 Teagan travelled by train to Truro.
4 Tim took until Tuesday to tidy his tools.
5 Tristan tripped over Troy's trick tricycle.

Odd word out – initial sounds

Involving words beginning with the 't' sound

→ The children are told which initial sound to listen for. They then listen while the teacher reads aloud one line of three words at a time. After each line the children are asked to say which word did not begin with the target sound.

1	tail	hen	tea
2	fire	tent	tie
3	toast	tongue	fork
4	drum	toe	tusk
5	two	thumb	teeth
6	pan	tap	ten
7	tall	tin	horn
8	torch	bench	tube
9	lick	tank	till
10	turkey	tiger	lucky
11	taxi	pixie	turnip
12	turn	touch	church
13	tortoise	puffin	tadpole
14	tomato	potato	television
15	flower	towel	table

Odd word out – rhyming
Using a word beginning with the 't' sound

→ The children are told to listen for the word that does not rhyme with the other two. They then listen while the teacher reads aloud one line of three words at a time. After each line the children are asked to say which word does not rhyme with the other two.

→ Alternatively, the children could be asked to say which two words do rhyme.

→ As an extra task, the children could think of other words that rhyme with the two rhyming words in each set.

1	pail	tail	lane
2	ten	man	hen
3	lap	weep	tap
4	torch	porch	beach
5	sent	net	tent
6	foal	hoe	toe
7	fin	tin	pen
8	till	wall	fill
9	barn	turn	churn
10	tank	pink	bank

Words to sound out for the 't' sound

→ Only words with regular spelling have been included.

→ The teacher takes one word at a time and 'sounds out' each phoneme. This may need to be done several times. The children must then guess what the word is. Some children may be able to try writing the word.

→ The children may like to repeat the phonemes consecutively, just as the teacher did, to help them blend the sounds into words.

t—e—n	t—a—p	t—ai—l	t—ee—th
t—e—n—t	t—u—s—k	t—ea	t—oa—s—t

Story for the 't' sound

→ The teacher asks the children to listen carefully to the story and pick out the words beginning with the target sound. The teacher then reads the story, sentence by sentence. After each sentence the teacher asks the children:

- To say how many words they heard beginning with the given sound in that sentence.
- To repeat the words they heard beginning with the target sound.

→ Alternatively, the teacher can slowly read the whole story, and the children can make a tally mark on a piece of paper every time they hear a word beginning with the target sound. The children can then count up how many words they have heard beginning with that sound and tell the teacher what those words are.

The wasted journey

Last Tuesday, Toby and Tyler went to see their friend, Todd. Todd lived in a town twenty miles away. To get there they had to take a bus to the station, a train and then another bus. The trip took them two hours. Toby and Tyler got off the second bus in Tennyson Road and looked for number twelve. Number twelve Tennyson Road was surrounded by trees. As they walked up the path, Toby and Tyler heard a terrible noise. It was Todd playing his tuba. Toby and Tyler touched the bell on the door. Todd's mum, Mrs Timothy, came to the door. She told them that Todd could not come out with them today because he had not tidied up his toys yet. Toby and Tyler said that they only wanted to talk to Todd. Toby and Tyler also promised to help Todd to tidy up his toys. Todd's mum told them that they would have to come back another time and that it might be better if they telephoned first. So Toby and Tyler turned round and started the two-hour journey back to Tollbridge, where they lived.

Puzzle worksheet for the 't' sound

Use the 't' pictures to help you with these puzzles.

Unscramble the words below. They all begin with 't'.

1 ttne   **2** btael   **3** getri   **4** eehtt   **5** ototam

_____   _____   _____   _____   _____

Look for the 't' words in the wordsearch below. They can read down or across. There are eight 't' words of three or more letters.

t	a	p	y	u	t	e	n
e	w	s	d	q	o	h	g
t	a	i	l	j	r	f	k
d	l	t	s	b	t	e	a
t	v	o	n	c	o	m	x
w	z	a	u	t	i	e	q
o	x	s	y	j	s	p	l
m	j	t	b	r	e	w	d

Write down the words that you found:

1 _____   **2** _____

3 _____   **4** _____

5 _____   **6** _____

7 _____   **8** _____

143

Illustrations for the 't' sound

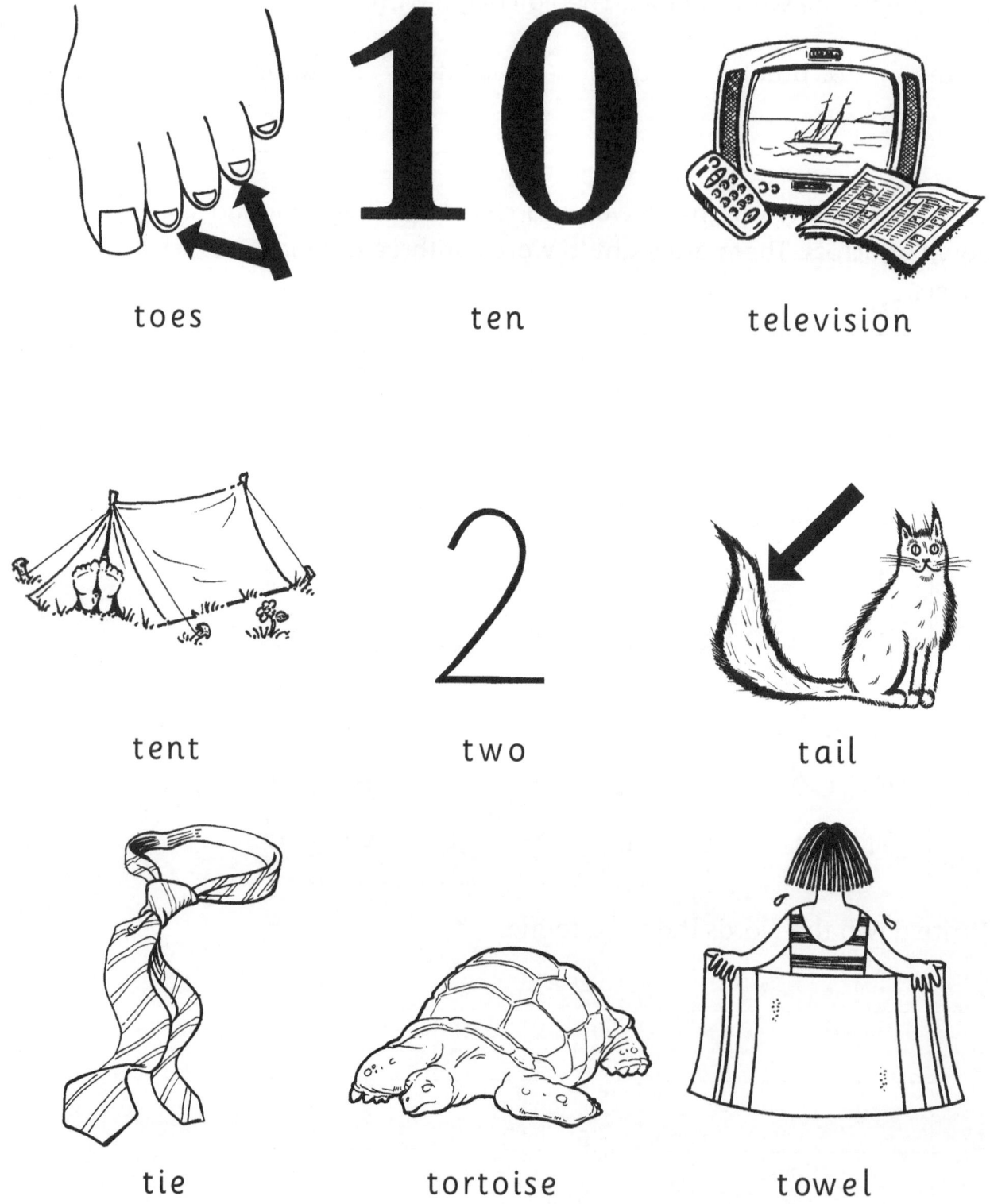

toes

10
ten

television

tent

2
two

tail

tie

tortoise

towel

Illustrations for the 't' sound

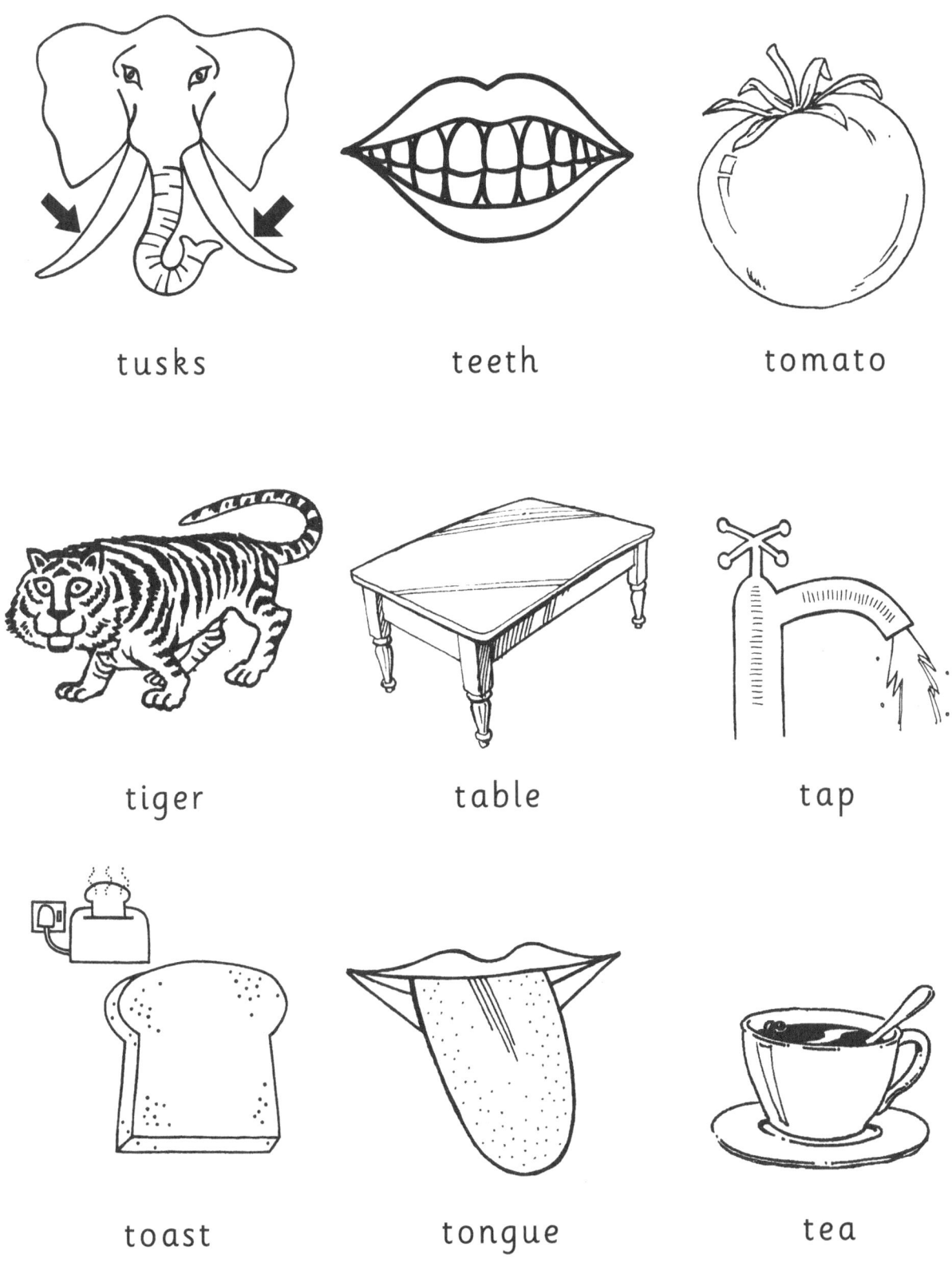

tusks

teeth

tomato

tiger

table

tap

toast

tongue

tea

Section for the 'v' and 'w' sounds

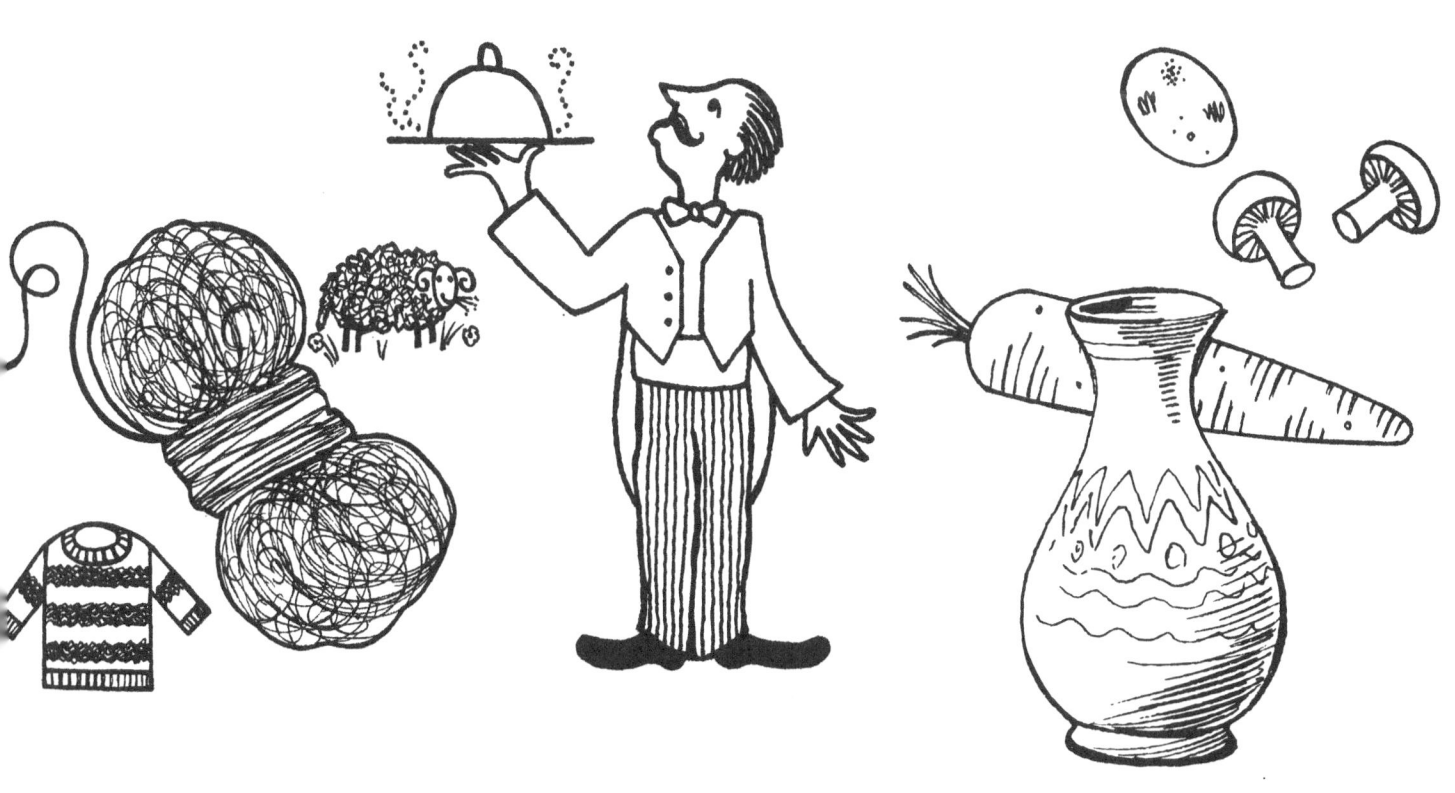

Section for the 'v' and 'w' sounds

Riddles for the 'v' and 'w' sounds

→ Children are given the photocopied pictures to go with the target sounds. The teacher reads out the riddles, one at a time, and the children decide which picture each one refers to. If desired, the children can then colour these pictures in.

→ *To make the activity more difficult*, the children, without access to the pictures, are told the target sounds, and the riddles are read out one at a time. The children have to think of something that starts with those sounds and fits in with the riddle.

→ *To teach vocabulary*, the teacher and the children look together at the photocopied pictures, and the teacher names and talks about each illustration. The teacher then proceeds to read out the riddles as suggested above.

1   Potatoes are one of these. Carrots are one. (*vegetables*)
2   It has strings. It makes music when you play it. (*violin*)
3   Spiders might spin one. They trap flies in it. (*web*)
4   It has a face. It has hands. (*watch*)
5   It is long and thin. You can use it to knit with. (*wool*)
6   It has no legs. It lives in the soil. (*worm*)
7   She wears black clothes. She wears a pointed hat. (*witch*)
8   You can open it and close it. It might have curtains in front of it. (*window*)
9   You put water in it. You put flowers in it. (*vase*)
10 It is covered in feathers. It is part of a bird. (*wing*)
11 It is wet. It comes out of a tap. (*water*)
12 It has four wheels. You can drive this. (*van*)

Alliteration for the 'v' and 'w' sounds

Suitable for children in Years R, 1 and 2

→ The teacher states what the target sounds are. They then read out each two-word phrase, and, after each one, the children must say whether one word or both words start with the target sounds.

→ Alternatively, the teacher can give each child two cards with the target sounds printed on. If both words in the phrase begin with one of the target sounds, the children hold up two cards. If only one begins with one of the target sounds, they hold up one card.

wicked witch	rough wool
wooden window	magic wand
warm kettle	windy weather
wild wolf	wise owl
vanilla custard	velvet curtains
cotton vest	violet vase

Tongue twisters for the 'v' and 'w' sounds

Suitable for children in Years R, 1 and 2

→ The teacher reads each tongue twister aloud and, after each one, asks the children to repeat it once or twice.

→ The children can play a game of Chinese Whispers. The teacher whispers the tongue twister to one child; this child whispers it to the next and so on. The last child says out loud what they think the teacher said, and this is compared with the original tongue twister.

1 Victor, the vampire, vanished in Virginia.
2 Viv visited Vicky in Vienna.
3 Vaughan varnished Valerie's valuable vase.
4 Wesley wanted a warm woolly waistcoat.
5 William wore wellies in the wet weather.

Odd word out — initial sounds

Involving words beginning with the 'v' and 'w' sounds

→ The children are told which initial sounds to listen for. They then listen while the teacher reads aloud one line of three words at a time. After each line the children are asked to say which word did not begin with one of the target sounds.

1	worm	lid	web
2	lap	wish	wing
3	witch	wolf	foal
4	well	farm	worm
5	wool	tool	watch
6	van	band	vase
7	vet	veil	dove
8	wall	wet	nought
9	send	wand	wig
10	water	otter	wider
11	finger	violin	vegetables
12	village	pillow	video
13	window	waiter	letter
14	baker	vicar	velvet
15	wardrobe	wizard	drawbridge

Odd word out — rhyming

Using a word beginning with the 'v' or 'w' sound

Suitable for children in Years R, 1 and 2

→ The children are told to listen for the word that does not rhyme with the other two. They then listen while the teacher reads aloud one line of three words at a time. After each line the children are asked to say which word does not rhyme with the other two.

→ Alternatively, the children could be asked to say which two words do rhyme.

→ As an extra task, the children could think of other words that rhyme with the two rhyming words in each set.

1	vest	hen	nest
2	pill	wool	bull
3	wall	crawl	seal
4	rest	tent	west
5	were	fur	car
6	wish	dish	pitch
7	tall	stale	veil
8	warm	farm	storm
9	lighter	daughter	water
10	vicar	flicker	cricket

Words to sound out for the 'v' and 'w' sounds

Suitable for children in Years R, 1 and 2

→ Only words with regular spelling have been included.

→ The teacher takes one word at a time and 'sounds out' each phoneme. This may need to be done several times. The children must then guess what the word is. Some children may be able to try writing the word.

→ The children may like to repeat the phonemes consecutively, just as the teacher did, to help them blend the sounds into words.

v—e—t	v—a—n	v—e—s—t	w—oo—l
w—i—sh	w—e—ll	w—oo—d	w—e—t

Stories for the 'v' and 'w' sounds

→ The teacher asks the children to listen carefully to the story and pick out the words beginning with the target sound. The teacher then reads the story, sentence by sentence. After each sentence the teacher asks the children:
  – To say how many words they heard beginning with the given sound in that sentence.
  – To repeat the words they heard beginning with the target sound.
→ Alternatively, the teacher can slowly read the whole story, and the children can make a tally mark on a piece of paper every time they hear a word beginning with the target sound. The children can then count up how many words they have heard beginning with that sound and tell the teacher what those words are.

Victoria's busy day ('v' sound)

Victoria had a busy day. First she took her cat, Virgil, to the vet's. Then she had a violin lesson with the vicar. After this, Victoria visited her friend Venus. Victoria and Venus decided to go shopping in the village. Venus' father, Vinny, gave them a lift in his van. Vinny parked the van near Vauxhall Station and arranged to meet Victoria and Venus at 4 o'clock. Venus bought a velvet dress for Val's party. Victoria bought five new vests and a blue vase for her mother. After shopping, Venus bought two vanilla ice-creams. Victoria and Venus met Vanessa and stopped to talk to her, forgetting the time. It was 5 o'clock and they were very late. When Victoria and Venus got to Vauxhall station, Vinny and his van had vanished. Victoria and Venus had a very long walk back to Venus' house.

1/2

Match postponed ('w' sound)

Wayne looked at his watch. His friend Wilf was late. Wayne and Wilf were going to watch the football match. Wolverhampton Wanderers were to play against Wallsend United at Willow Road football ground. Wayne decided to walk to Willow Road by himself. As it was wet, cold and windy, Wayne wore his Wellington boots and warm coat. Wayne walked down Water Lane and turned left into Wicker Road. It was raining fast, and Wayne's clothes felt wet. As he reached Willow Road football ground, Wayne saw a notice. It said, 'Due to a waterlogged pitch the match will now take place on Wednesday evening.' A very wet Wayne walked to Wilf's house and knocked on the door. Mrs Willis answered the door and said that Wilf had got wet walking home from work and had fallen asleep by the fire. Mrs Willis had not wanted to wake Wilf up. However, Mrs Willis saw how wet Wayne was so she asked him into the kitchen and gave him a warm drink. Then Mrs Willis put Wayne's wet clothes in the washing machine. She gave Wayne some of Wilf's clothes to walk home in.

Puzzle worksheet for 'v' and 'w' sounds

Use the 'v' and 'w' pictures to help you with these puzzles.

Unscramble the words below. They all begin with 'v' or 'w'.

1 anv   **2** svte   **3** chitw   **4** aewtr   **5** cwhat

_____   _____   _____   _____   _____

Look for the 'v' and 'w' words in the wordsearch below. They can read down or across. There are eight 'v' or 'w' words of three letters or more.

v	a	s	e	w	s	g	t
i	b	g	y	i	x	n	w
o	m	w	z	n	c	r	i
l	u	a	p	g	v	a	n
i	k	l	v	h	f	j	d
n	g	l	e	b	q	r	o
t	n	p	s	s	f	d	w
f	w	i	t	c	h	s	u

Write down the words that you found:

1 _____   2 _____

3 _____   4 _____

5 _____   6 _____

7 _____   8 _____

Illustrations for the 'v' and 'w' sounds

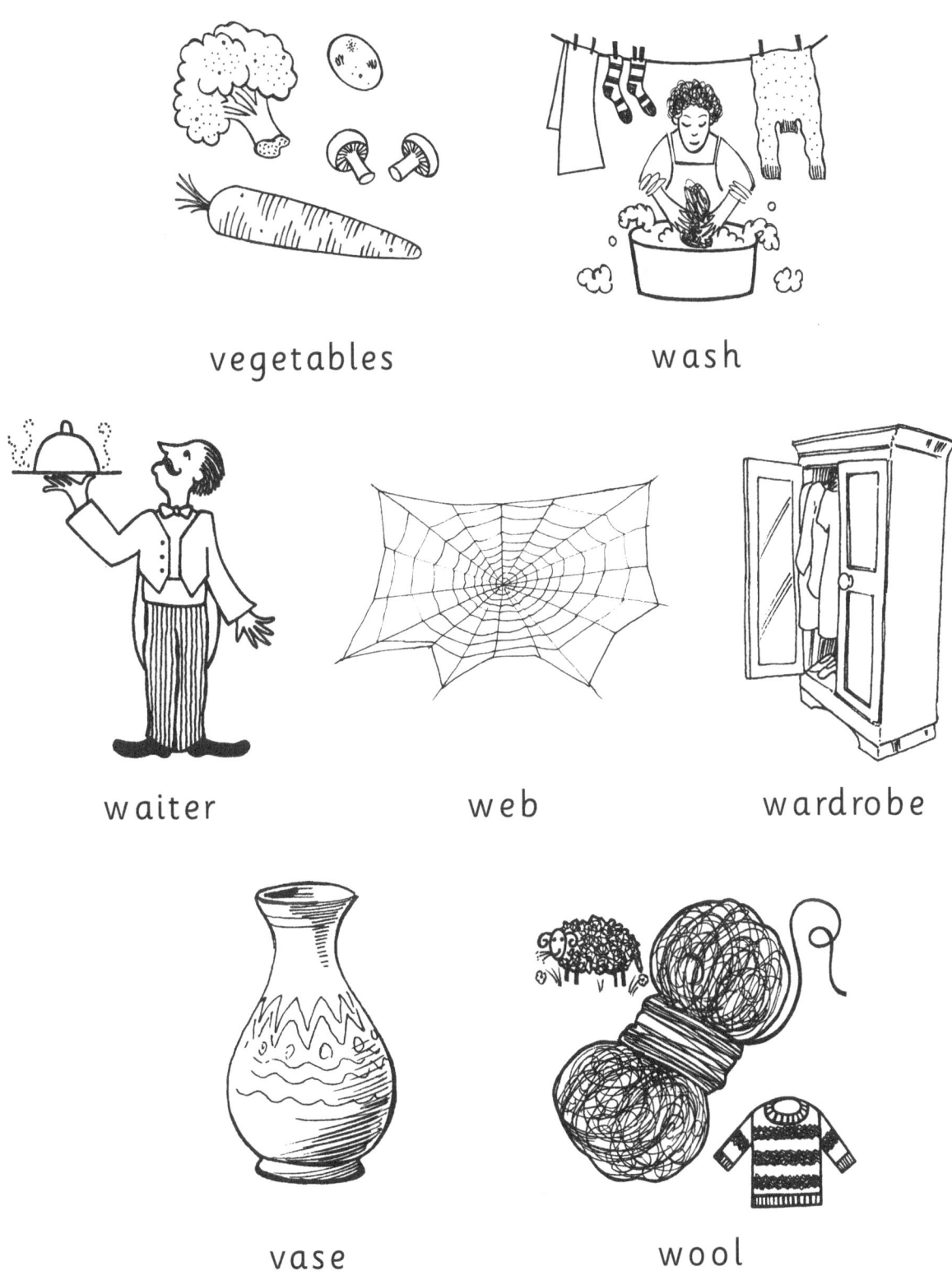

vegetables

wash

waiter

web

wardrobe

vase

wool

1/3

Illustrations for the 'v' and 'w' sounds

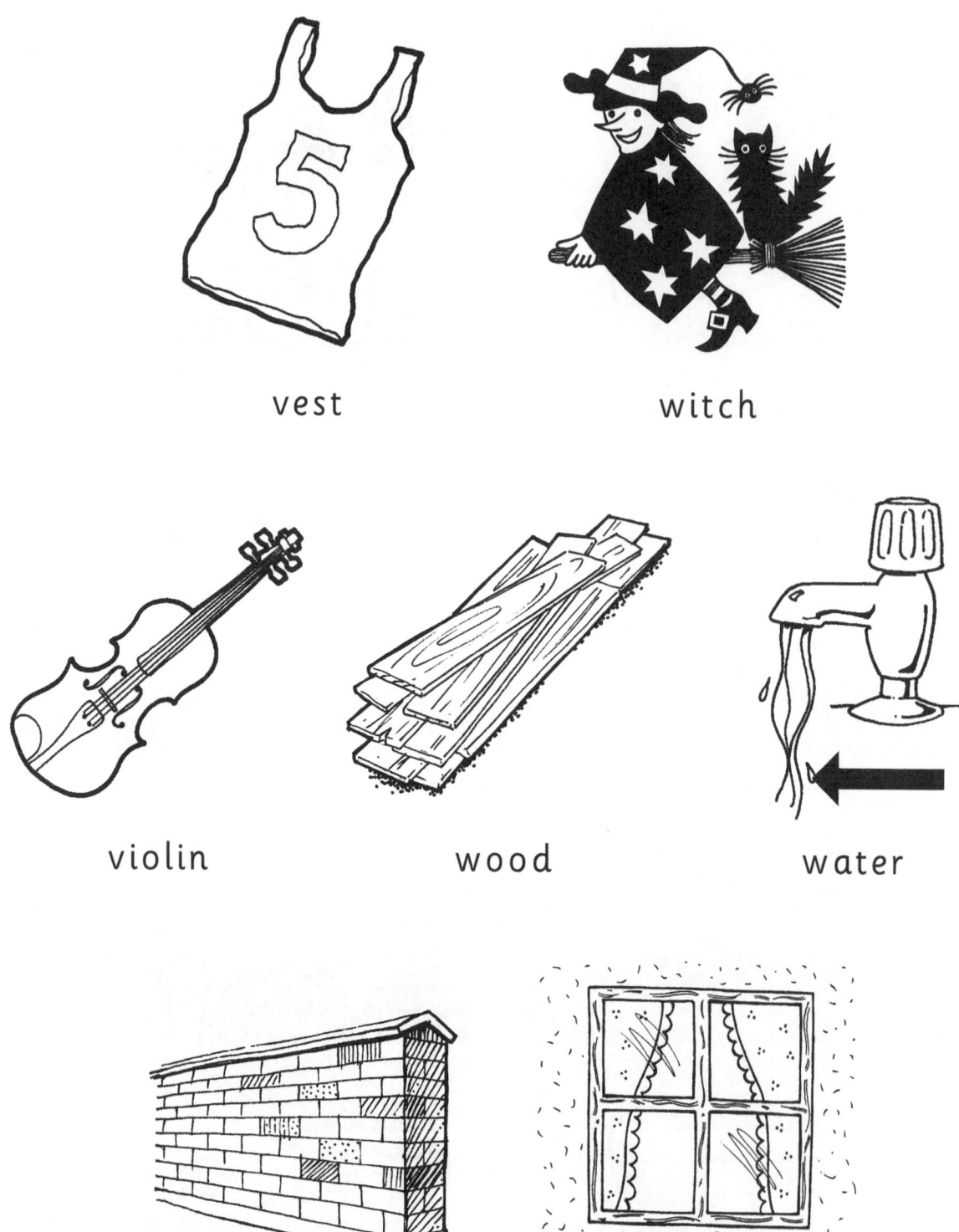

vest

witch

violin

wood

water

wall

window

Illustrations for the 'v' and 'w' sounds

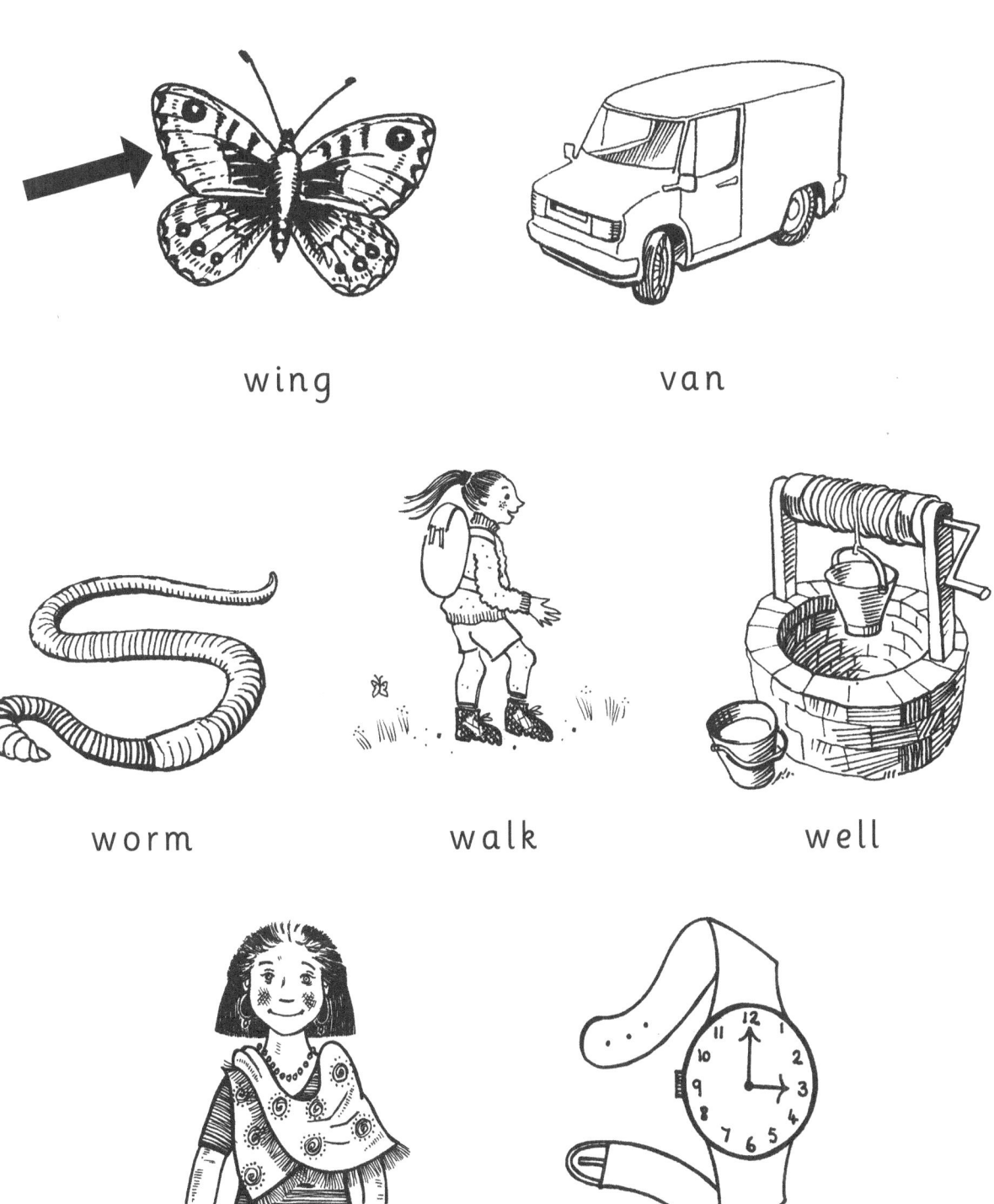

wing

van

worm

walk

well

woman

watch

3/3

Routledge
Taylor & Francis Group

Section for the 'y' and 'th' (unvoiced) sounds

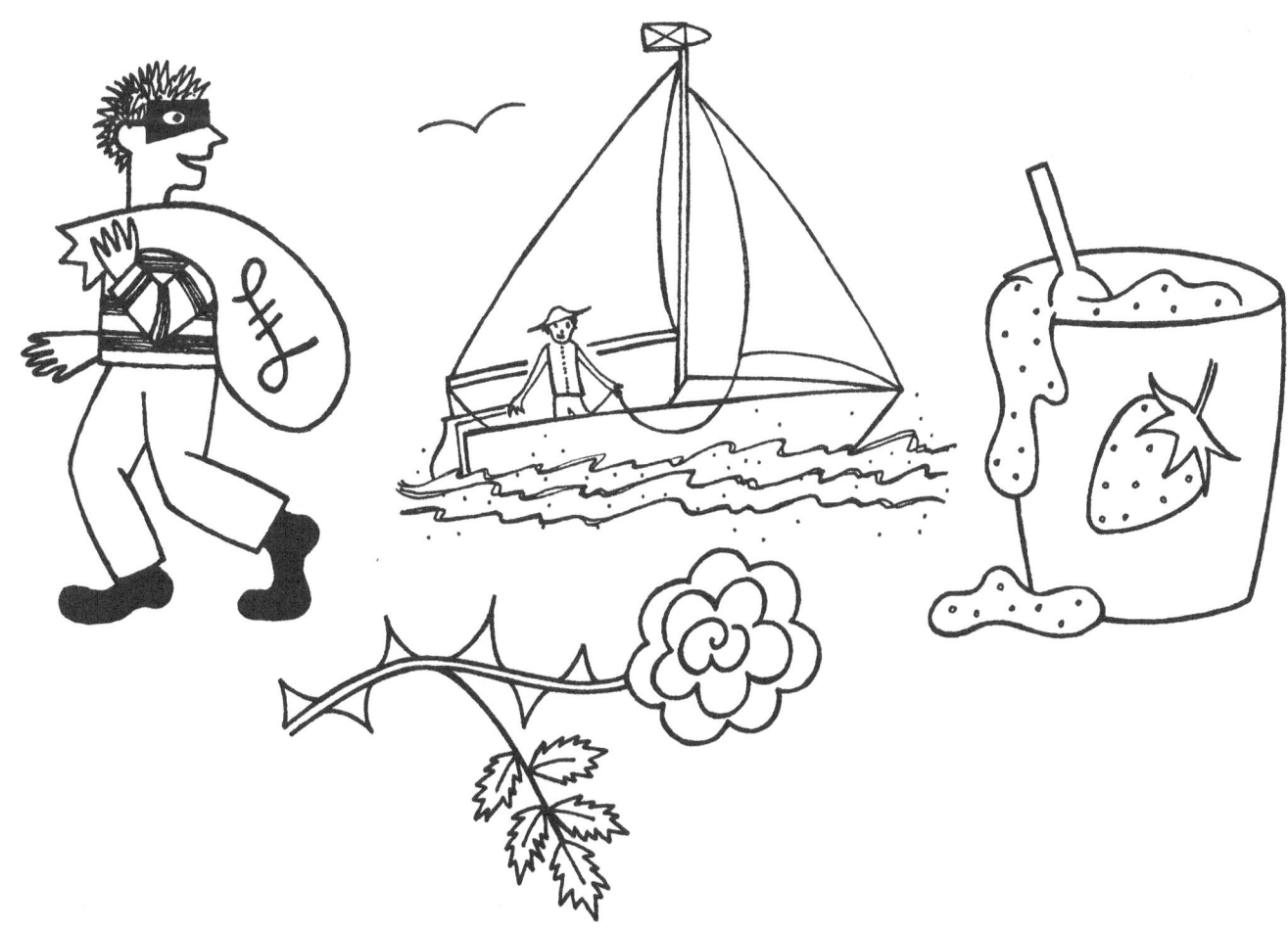

Section for the 'y' and 'th' (unvoiced) sounds

Riddles for the 'y' and 'th' sounds

→ Children are given the photocopied pictures to go with the target sounds. The teacher reads out the riddles, one at a time, and the children decide which picture each one refers to. If desired, the children can then colour these pictures in.

→ *To make the activity more difficult*, the children, without access to the pictures, are told the target sounds, and the riddles are read out one at a time. The children have to think of something that starts with those sounds and fits in with the riddle.

→ *To teach vocabulary*, the teacher and the children look together at the photocopied pictures, and the teacher names and talks about each illustration. The teacher then proceeds to read out the riddles as suggested above.

1 You play with it. It goes up and down. (*yo-yo*)
2 It is a part of your body. It is joined to your hand. (*thumb*)
3 This is a number. It is one less than four. (*three*)
4 You might find this on a rose stem. It might prick you. (*thorn*)
5 This is someone who breaks the law. They steal things. (*thief*)
6 You can eat this. It is the middle of an egg. (*yolk*)
7 This is part of your body. It is under your chin. (*throat*)
8 You can eat this. It is made with milk. (*yogurt*)
9 This can be lots of different colours. You can sew with it. (*thread*)
10 This is a number. It comes after twelve. (*thirteen*)
11 You might see one on the sea. It usually has two sails. (*yacht*)
12 It is like a chair. A king or queen might sit on one. (*throne*)

Alliteration for the 'y' and 'th' sounds

→ The teacher states what the target sounds are. They then read out each two-word phrase, and, after each one, the children must say whether one word or both words start with the target sounds.

→ Alternatively, the teacher can give each child two cards with the target sounds printed on. If both words in the phrase begin with one of the target sounds, the children hold up two cards. If only one begins with one of the target sounds, they hold up one card.

thick wool	thin pencil
sharp thorn	three thrushes
throbbing throat	thorny thistles
yappy dog	two years
tall yacht	young yak
strawberry yogurt	yellow yolk

Tongue twisters for the 'y' and 'th' sounds

→ The teacher reads each tongue twister aloud and, after each one, asks the children to repeat it once or twice.

→ The children can play a game of Chinese Whispers. The teacher whispers the tongue twister to one child; this child whispers it to the next and so on. The last child says out loud what they think the teacher said, and this is compared with the original tongue twister.

1 Thurston and Thora saw thirteen thrushes on Thursday.
2 Theodore had three thousand and thirty thermometers.
3 The thirsty thief's throat throbbed.
4 The youth yanked at Yasmin's yo-yo.
5 The young yak ate the yellow yogurt.

Odd word out — initial sounds

Involving words beginning with the 'y' and 'th' sounds

→ The children are told which initial sounds to listen for. They then listen while the teacher reads aloud one line of three words at a time. After each line the children are asked to say which word did not begin with the target sound.

1	sing	thin	think
2	three	throw	saw
3	thorn	thief	fox
4	thumb	jump	thick
5	chalk	thank	thought
6	street	thread	throat
7	yolk	cone	yawn
8	yak	you	juice
9	doll	yacht	yell
10	thaw	fourth	thigh
11	panda	thunder	thicker
12	throne	born	throb
13	thirteen	thistle	castle
14	cherry	thirty	Thursday
15	yogurt	joker	yo-yo

162

Odd word out — rhyming
Using a word beginning with the 'y' or 'th' sound

→ The children are told to listen for the word that does not rhyme with the other two. They then listen while the teacher reads aloud one line of three words at a time. After each line the children are asked to say which word does not rhyme with the other two.

→ Alternatively, the children could be asked to say which two words do rhyme.

→ As an extra task, the children could think of other words that rhyme with the two rhyming words in each set.

1	thorn	horn	barn
2	thief	feet	leaf
3	fat	throat	coat
4	thumb	mud	hum
5	forty	dirty	thirty
6	thread	bed	food
7	three	four	sea
8	yolk	woke	coal
9	chalk	yak	pack
10	yacht	wet	cot

Words to sound out for the 'y' and 'th' sounds

→ Only words with regular spelling have been included.

→ The teacher takes one word at a time and 'sounds out' each phoneme. This may need to be done several times. The children must then guess what the word is. Some children may be able to try writing the word.

→ The children may like to repeat the phonemes consecutively, just as the teacher did, to help them blend the sounds into words.

th—or—n	th—i—ck	y—aw—n	th—r—ee
y—a—k	th—r—u—sh	th—r—oa—t	th—i—n

Stories for the 'y' and 'th' sounds

→ The teacher asks the children to listen carefully to the story and pick out the words beginning with the target sound. The teacher then reads the story, sentence by sentence. After each sentence the teacher asks the children:

- To say how many words they heard beginning with the given sound in that sentence.
- To repeat the words they heard beginning with the target sound.

→ Alternatively, the teacher can slowly read the whole story, and the children can make a tally mark on a piece of paper every time they hear a word beginning with the target sound. The children can then count up how many words they have heard beginning with that sound and tell the teacher what those words are.

Yasmin's cat ('y' sound)

Yasmin had a young cat called Yummy, who liked to play with yo-yos. Yasmin would make the yo-yo go up and down while Yummy tried to catch it. One day Yummy yelped, jumped up high and knocked a yellow bowl off the table. The eggs in the bowl fell out, and the yolks broke as they hit the floor. Yummy licked up some of the yolks. Yasmin yelled at Yummy to get out of the way. Yummy jumped up on the shelf and knocked off a little china yacht. Yasmin then noticed something yellow on the floor. Yasmin picked it up. It was a ring that Yasmin had lost a year ago. Yasmin was so pleased to find her yellow ring that she gave Yummy some of his favourite yogurt.

1/2

The little thrush ('th' sound)

Theo, Thornton and Thackery were throwing stones at a thrush. The little thrush hopped through the thick hedge. The three boys tried to get through the hedge after the thrush. Theo pricked his thumb on a thorn and cried because it throbbed. Thackery scratched his throat on a thistle, and Thornton cut his thigh on a sharp stone. Mrs Thrower, who lived in the house with the hedge, saw the frightened thrush. She guessed that the three boys had been throwing things at it. Mrs Thrower found a thick towel and placed the thrush in it. Thankfully, after 30 minutes, the thrush recovered, and flew away. A week later the three boys were coming home from school during a thunderstorm. Theo, Thackery and Thornton were afraid of thunder. Just as the three boys were passing Mrs Thrower's hedge, there was a very loud clap of thunder. The three boys dived under Mrs Thrower's hedge. Theo, Thackery and Thornton must have disturbed some thrushes' nests. The three boys found themselves being attacked by three thrushes who were trying to protect their babies. They thrashed about trying to throw off the thrushes. In the end the three boys managed to throw off the thrushes and escape. Theo, Thackery and Thornton had learned their lesson, and they never harmed a thrush or any other creature again.

2/2

165

Puzzle worksheet for 'y' and 'th' sounds

Use the 'y' and 'th' pictures to help you with these puzzles.

Unscramble the words below. They all begin with 'y' or 'th'.

1 aynw   **2** okly   **3** tubmh   **4** otnhr   **5** rhete

_____   _____   _____   _____   _____

Look for the 'y' and 'th' words in the wordsearch below. They can read down or across. There are eight 'y' or 'th' words of three letters or more.

w	t	h	o	r	n	y	r
g	h	k	p	u	d	a	t
t	r	y	o	l	k	c	h
h	e	x	c	v	b	h	r
r	a	z	s	d	f	t	e
o	d	q	y	a	w	n	e
a	e	j	w	y	z	k	g
t	x	t	h	u	m	b	u

Write down the words that you found:

1 _____   2 _____

3 _____   4 _____

5 _____   6 _____

7 _____   8 _____

Illustrations for the 'y' and 'th' sounds

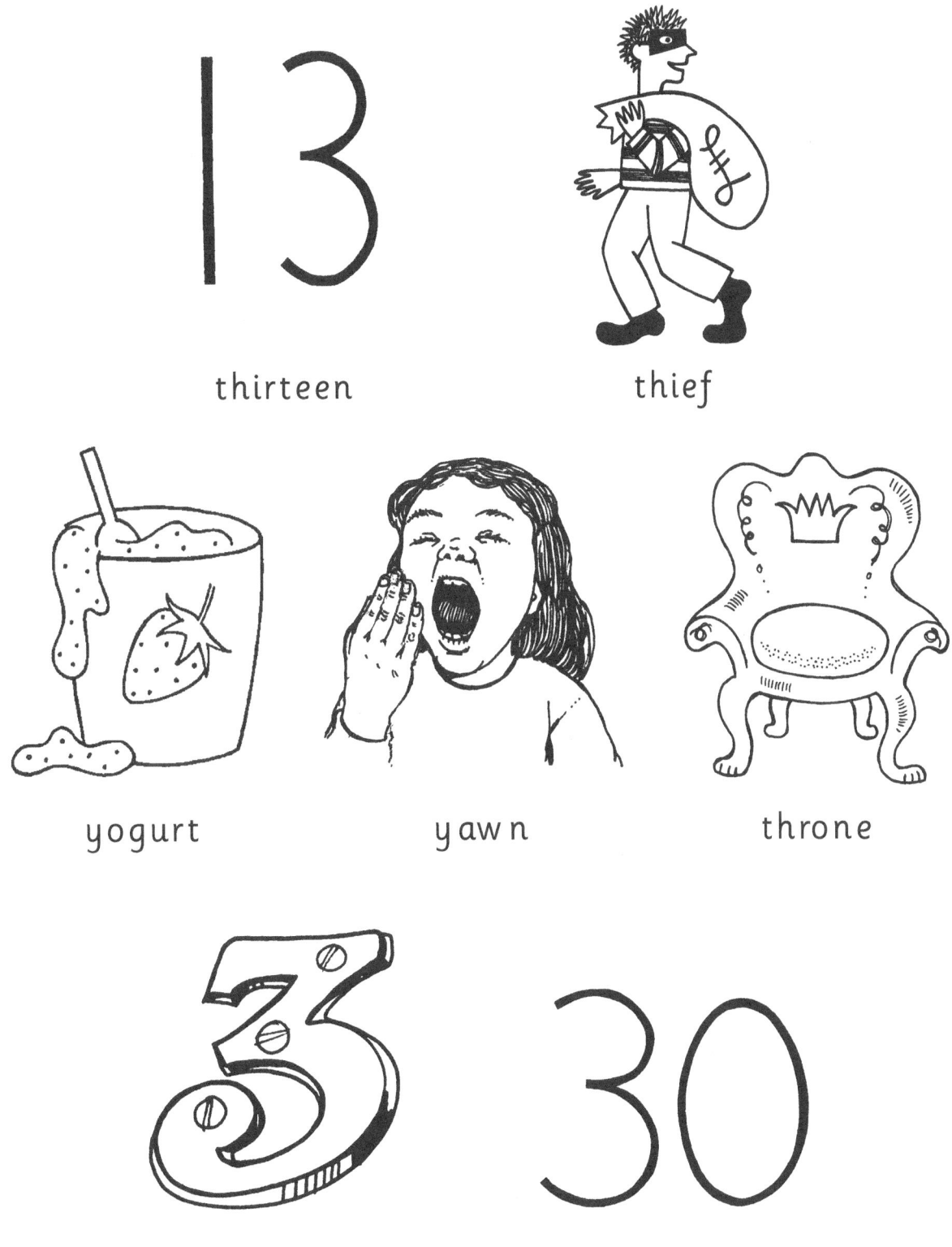

thirteen   thief

yogurt   yawn   throne

three   thirty

1/2

Illustrations for the 'y' and 'th' sounds

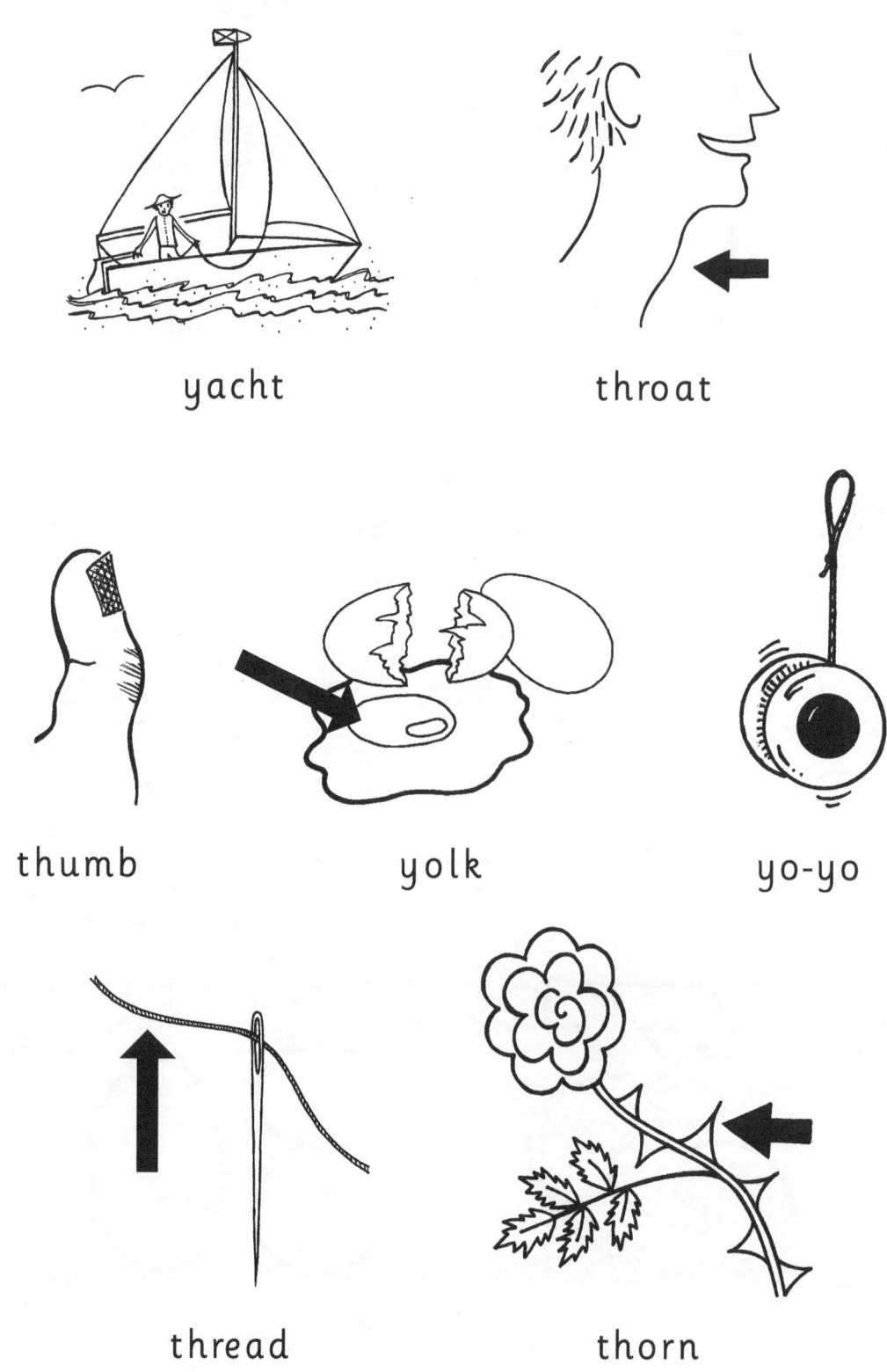

yacht

throat

thumb

yolk

yo-yo

thread

thorn

Section for the 'sh' sound

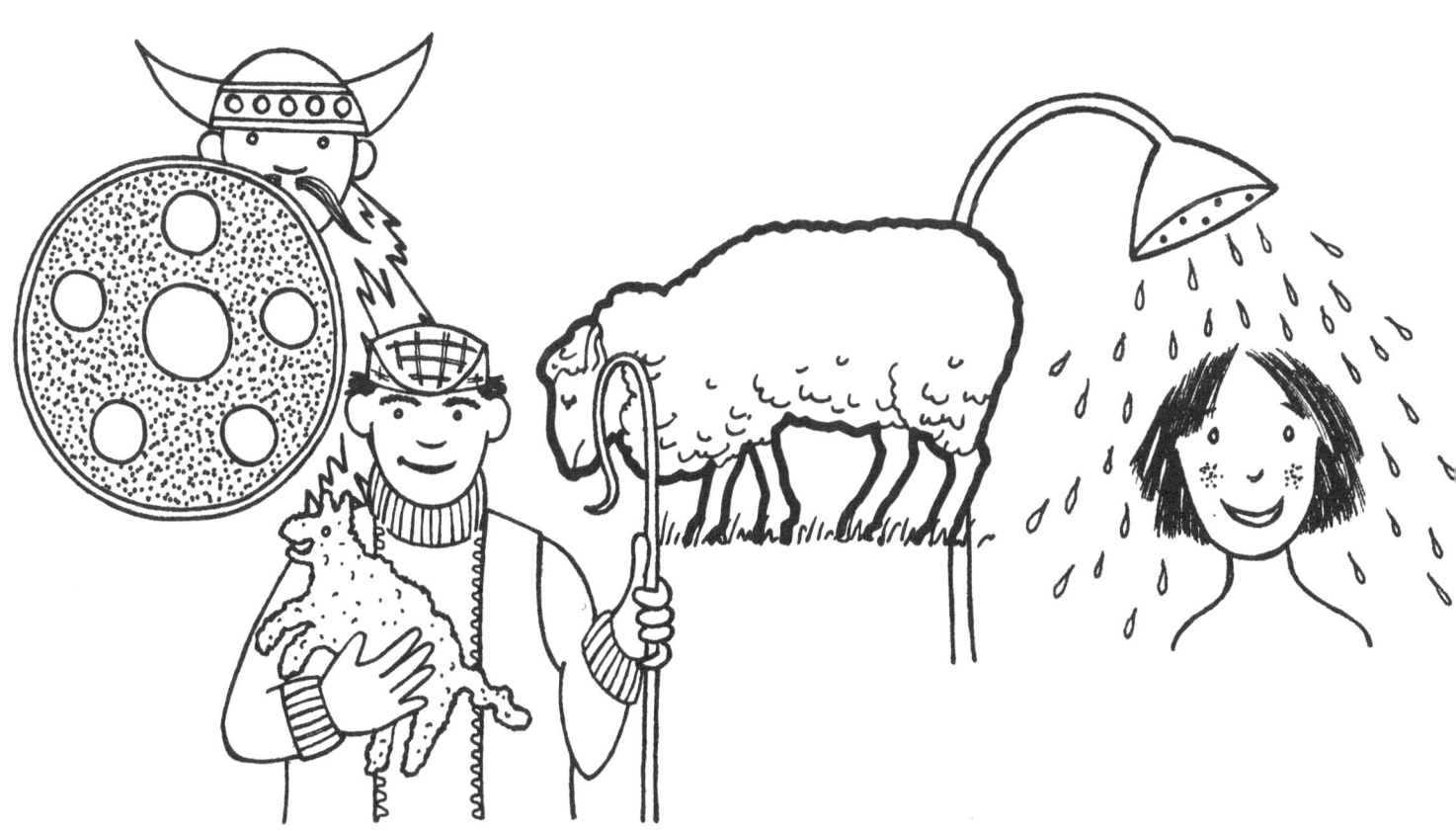

Section for the 'sh' sound

Riddles for the 'sh' sound

→ Children are given the photocopied pictures to go with the target sound. The teacher reads out the riddles, one at a time, and the children decide which picture each one refers to. If desired, the children can then colour these pictures in.

→ *To make the activity more difficult*, the children, without access to the pictures, are told the target sound, and the riddles are read out one at a time. The children have to think of something that starts with that sound and fits in with the riddle.

→ *To teach vocabulary*, the teacher and the children look together at the photocopied pictures, and the teacher names and talks about each illustration. The teacher then proceeds to read out the riddles as suggested above.

1 It is made or wood or metal. You can put things on it. (*shelf*)
2 It is part of your body. It is at the top of your arm. (*shoulder*)
3 You might have one in the bathroom. Water comes out of it. (*shower*)
4 They have legs. You wear them. (*shorts*)
5 It can be fierce. It has a big fin on its back. (*shark*)
6 It has buttons. It has a collar. (*shirt*)
7 It has a heel. You wear it on your foot. (*shoe*)
8 It has a door and is usually made of wood. You might have one in your garden. (*shed*)
9 It has four legs. It has a woolly coat in the winter. (*sheep*)
10 This is a liquid. You put it on your hair. (*shampoo*)
11 It is very big. It sails on the sea. (*ship*)
12 A tortoise has one. A snail has one. (*shell*)

Alliteration for the 'sh' sound

Suitable for children in Years R, 1 and 2

→ The teacher states what the target sound is. They then read out each two-word phrase, and, after each one, the children must say whether one word or both words start with the target sound.

→ Alternatively, the teacher can give each child two cards with the target sound printed on. If both words in the phrase begin with the target sound, the children hold up two cards. If only one begins with that sound, they hold up one card.

sharp shell	garden shed
shiny shoes	coloured shirt
toy shop	shaking shepherd
shopping trolley	short street
woolly sheep	shoe shop
shy shark	frothy shampoo

Tongue twisters for the 'sh' sound

Suitable for children in Years R, 1 and 2

→ The teacher reads each tongue twister aloud and, after each one, asks the children to repeat it once or twice.

→ The children can play a game of Chinese Whispers. The teacher whispers the tongue twister to one child; this child whispers it to the next and so on. The last child says out loud what they think the teacher said, and this is compared with the original tongue twister.

1 The shocked shark shivered in the shipwreck.
2 Sheryl sheared the shaking sheep.
3 Shelley should shorten the chef's shirt.
4 Shaun shifted the shiny shoes onto the shelf.
5 The shrews shrieked at the shrivelled shrimps.

Odd word out — initial sounds

Involving words beginning with the 'sh' sound

→ The children are told which initial sound to listen for. They then listen while the teacher reads aloud one line of three words at a time. After each line the children are asked to say which word did not begin with the target sound.

1	ship	toad	sheet
2	shout	jump	show
3	brush	shelf	shop
4	shell	shoe	spoon
5	chick	shed	sheep
6	shark	shirt	dish
7	shorts	sweets	shield
8	shoot	shut	cheat
9	thaw	share	shy
10	show	cone	shine
11	hope	shape	sharp
12	shampoo	scarecrow	shepherd
13	yellow	shadow	shallow
14	shoulder	shovel	cover
15	shiny	trifle	shuffle

Odd word out – rhyming
Using a word beginning with the 'sh' sound

Suitable for children in Years R, 1 and 2

➜ The children are told to listen for the word that does not rhyme with the other two. They then listen while the teacher reads aloud one line of three words at a time. After each line the children are asked to say which word does not rhyme with the other two.

➜ Alternatively, the children could be asked to say which two words do rhyme.

➜ As an extra task, the children could think of other words that rhyme with the two rhyming words in each set.

1	shark	bark	peg
2	scarf	shed	bed
3	ship	rain	hip
4	foot	sheet	wheat
5	shoe	two	hoot
6	sheep	lip	deep
7	cap	shop	top
8	shell	bell	fall
9	crawled	shield	field
10	shower	towel	flower

Words to sound out for the 'sh' sound

Suitable for children in Years R, 1 and 2

➜ Only words with regular spelling have been included.

➜ The teacher takes one word at a time and 'sounds out' each phoneme. This may need to be done several times. The children must then guess what the word is. Some children may be able to try writing the word.

➜ The children may like to repeat the phonemes consecutively, just as the teacher did, to help them blend the sounds into words.

sh—ee—p	sh—ee—t	sh—i—p	sh—e—d
sh—o—p	sh—e—ll	sh—ar—k	sh—or—t

Story for the 'sh' sound

→ The teacher asks the children to listen carefully to the story and pick out the words beginning with the target sound. The teacher then reads the story, sentence by sentence. After each sentence the teacher asks the children:

- To say how many words they heard beginning with the given sound in that sentence.
- To repeat the words they heard beginning with the target sound.

→ Alternatively, the teacher can slowly read the whole story, and the children can make a tally mark on a piece of paper every time they hear a word beginning with the target sound. The children can then count up how many words they have heard beginning with that sound and tell the teacher what those words are.

Two showers in one day

Sherry had a shower and shampooed her hair. Then she put on her shirt, shorts, shoes and jacket. Carrying her trainers, she dashed out of the door, shutting it with a bang. It was a short walk down Shore Street to the bus stop. On the way, she stopped at the shop to buy some shortcake biscuits for Shane and herself to share. Shane was her elder brother, and she was to meet him at the gym. Shane had a job, to pay for his car, stacking shelves at Sharp's supermarket in Shelton. Sherry stood shivering in the bus shelter and waited for the bus from Shadwell to Shelton Town. As Sherry got off the bus at Shelton Town, there was a short, sharp shower of rain. Her shorts were soaked, and the water droplets trickled down her shins. Sherry was shaking with the cold when she reached the gym. She tried to open the gym door, but it was firmly shut. Just then she heard Shane shouting at her. She looked over her shoulder and saw Shane running up to the gym door. He showed Sherry the notice. It said, 'We apologise but we had to shut early due to being short of staff'. Luckily, Shane's shiny red car was parked in Sharp's car park nearby. Sherry did not have to wait in a draughty bus shelter for a bus back to Shadwell.

Puzzle worksheet for the 'sh' sound

Use the 'sh' pictures to help you with these puzzles.

Unscramble the words below. They all begin with 'sh'.

1 asrkh   **2** tihrs   **3** fhles   **4** ssorth   **5** lelhs

_____   _____   _____   _____   _____

Look for the 'sh' words in the wordsearch below. They can read down or across. There are eight 'sh' words of three letters or more.

r	s	h	o	p	o	n	b
a	c	f	s	h	e	e	p
s	h	a	m	p	o	o	k
s	d	g	j	l	f	x	s
h	z	c	s	w	b	r	h
e	p	s	h	e	d	a	i
l	t	y	o	u	k	n	p
l	s	h	e	l	f	j	c

Write down the words that you found:

1 _____   2 _____

3 _____   4 _____

5 _____   6 _____

7 _____   8 _____

175

Illustrations for the 'sh' sound

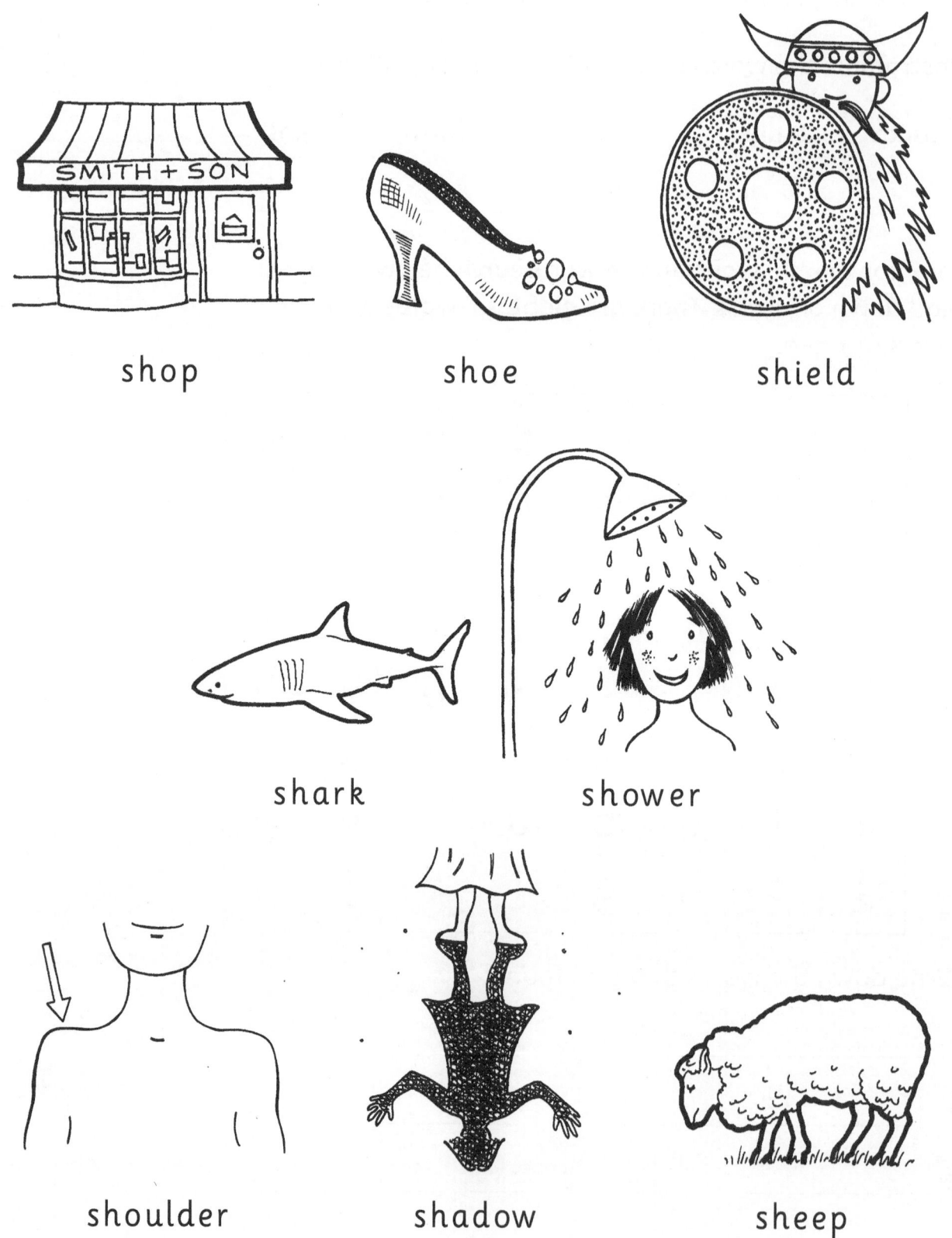

shop

shoe

shield

shark

shower

shoulder

shadow

sheep

Illustrations for the 'sh' sound

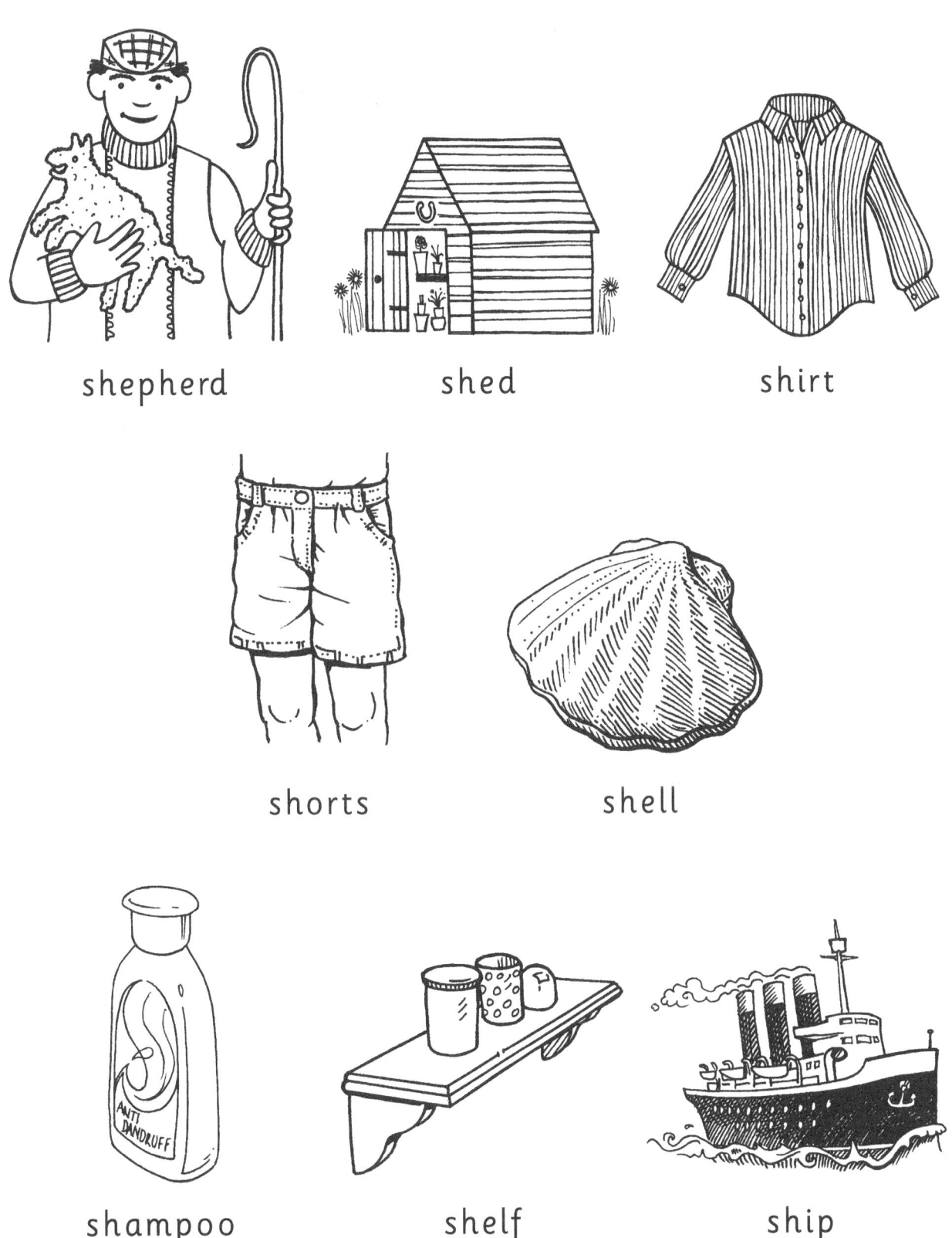

shepherd

shed

shirt

shorts

shell

shampoo

ANTI DANDRUFF

shelf

ship

2/2

Section for the 'ch' sound

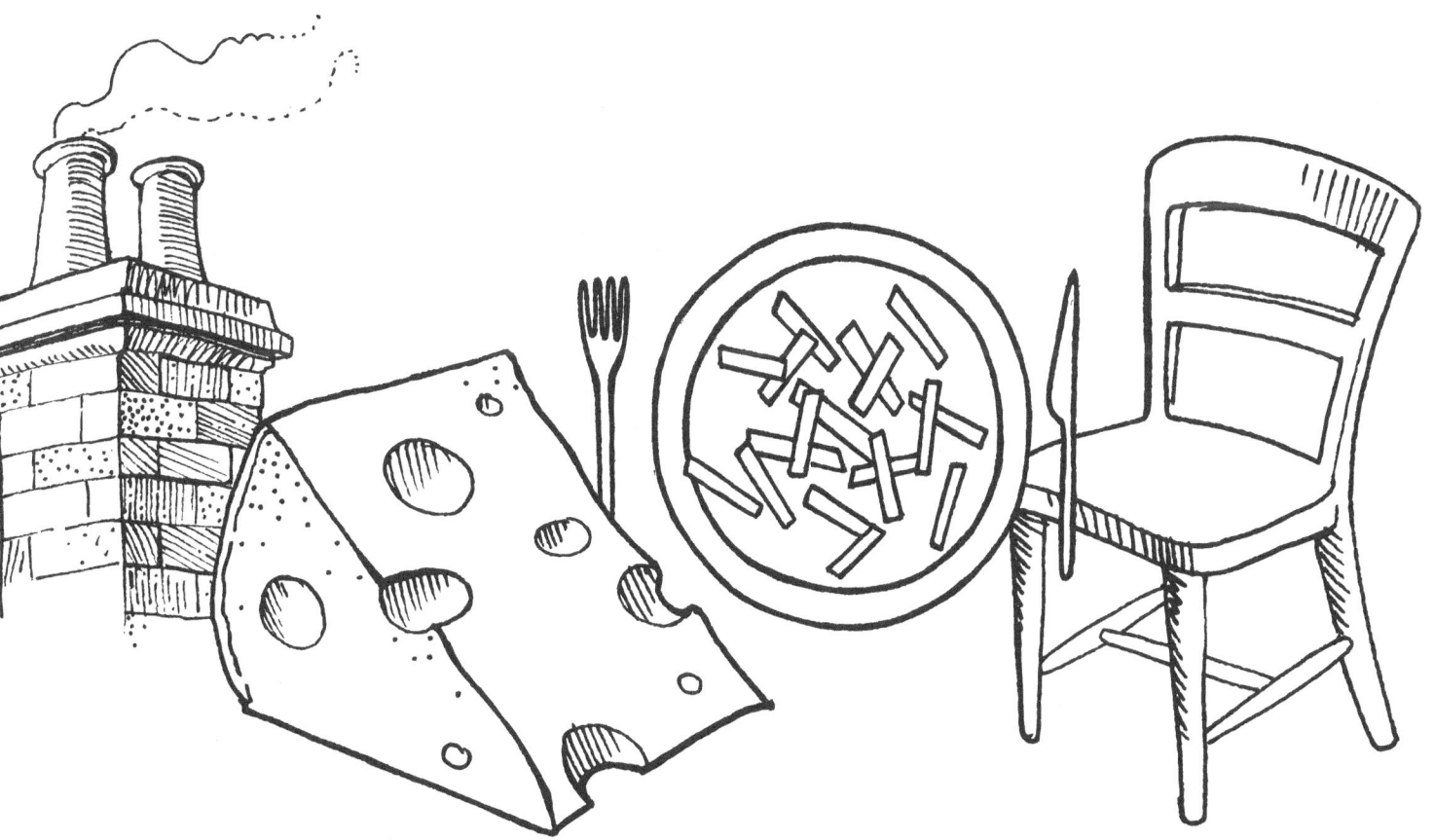

Section for the 'ch' sound

Riddles for the 'ch' sound

→ Children are given the photocopied pictures to go with the target sound. The teacher reads out the riddles, one at a time, and the children decide which picture each one refers to. If desired, the children can then colour these pictures in.

→ *To make the activity more difficult*, the children, without access to the pictures, are told the target sound, and the riddles are read out one at a time. The children have to think of something that starts with that sound and fits in with the riddle.

→ *To teach vocabulary*, the teacher and the children look together at the photocopied pictures, and the teacher names and talks about each illustration. The teacher then proceeds to read out the riddles as suggested above.

1 It is part of your face. It is under your eye. (*cheek*)
2 You can eat it. It is brown and sweet. (*chocolate*)
3 Smoke comes out of it. A house might have one on its roof. (*chimney*)
4 You can eat them. They are made from potatoes. (*chips*)
5 It has four legs. It has a back and it might have arms. (*chair*)
6 Pirates sometimes have one. They put treasure in it. (*chest*)
7 It can be white or coloured. You can draw or write with it. (*chalk*)
8 It has windows. It might have a tower or steeple. (*church*)
9 You can eat it. It has a stone in the middle. (*cherry*)
10 It has fluffy feathers. It is a baby. (*chick*)
11 It is part of your face. It is below your mouth. (*chin*)
12 You can eat it. It is made from milk. (*cheese*)

Alliteration for the 'ch' sound

Suitable for children in Years R, 1 and 2

→ The teacher states what the target sound is. They then read out each two-word phrase, and, after each one, the children must say whether one word or both words start with the target sound.

→ Alternatively, the teacher can give each child two cards with the target sound printed on. If both words in the phrase begin with the target sound, the children hold up two cards. If only one begins with that sound, they hold up one card.

cheerful chimp	sharp chisel
cheese pie	chocolate cheesecake
chatty chipmunks	cherry tart
chilly church	charming chick
choppy ocean	cheap chain
cheeky children	tall chimney

Tongue twisters for the 'ch' sound

Suitable for children in Years R, 1 and 2

→ The teacher reads each tongue twister aloud and, after each one, asks the children to repeat it once or twice.

→ The children can play a game of Chinese Whispers. The teacher whispers the tongue twister to one child; this child whispers it to the next and so on. The last child says out loud what they think the teacher said, and this is compared with the original tongue twister.

1 Charity had chocolate all over her chin and chubby cheeks.
2 The cheerful children chased the cheeky chipmunks.
3 Charlie chuckled at the cheetah chasing the chickens.
4 Cherry chose chopped chicken, chips and cheese.
5 Cheryl choked on her Chinese chicken and chestnuts.

Odd word out — initial sounds

Involving words beginning with the 'ch' sound

→ The children are told which initial sound to listen for. They then listen while the teacher reads aloud one line of three words at a time. After each line the children are asked to say which word did not begin with the target sound.

1	thigh	chin	chain
2	chair	sad	chalk
3	chop	chase	shawl
4	judge	cheek	cheese
5	chest	chick	drum
6	church	cap	chip
7	cheap	team	cheat
8	churn	chess	purse
9	cherry	chimney	tractor
10	ostrich	choppy	chilly
11	butcher	chocolate	children
12	letter	chapel	chatter
13	chaffinch	finger	chipmunk
14	chisel	china	thistle
15	chapter	after	cheerful

Odd word out – rhyming
Using a word beginning with the 'ch' sound

→ The children are told to listen for the word that does not rhyme with the other two. They then listen while the teacher reads aloud one line of three words at a time. After each line the children are asked to say which word does not rhyme with the other two.

→ Alternatively, the children could be asked to say which two words do rhyme.

→ As an extra task, the children could think of other words that rhyme with the two rhyming words in each set.

1	chalk	walk	fish
2	hot	chest	west
3	cheese	niece	sneeze
4	chain	gate	train
5	chair	deer	bear
6	church	birch	march
7	cheek	sheep	week
8	shin	sing	chin
9	marry	cherry	ferry
10	chilly	jolly	hilly

Words to sound out for the 'ch' sound

→ Only words with regular spelling have been included.

→ The teacher takes one word at a time and 'sounds out' each phoneme. This may need to be done several times. The children must then guess what the word is. Some children may be able to try writing the word.

→ The children may like to repeat the phonemes consecutively, just as the teacher did, to help them blend the sounds into words.

ch—ee—k	ch—i—n	ch—i—ck	ch—e—s—t
ch—i—p	ch—ai—n	ch—ur—ch	ch—ur—n

Story for the 'ch' sound

→ The teacher asks the children to listen carefully to the story and pick out the words beginning with the target sound. The teacher then reads the story, sentence by sentence. After each sentence the teacher asks the children:

    – To say how many words they heard beginning with the given sound in that sentence.

    – To repeat the words they heard beginning with the target sound.

→ Alternatively, the teacher can slowly read the whole story, and the children can make a tally mark on a piece of paper every time they hear a word beginning with the target sound. The children can then count up how many words they have heard beginning with that sound and tell the teacher what those words are.

Charlie the chimpanzee

Cheeky Charlie was a chimpanzee. One day Mr Chester, Charlie's keeper, left the cage door open so Charlie escaped. He saw a child eating a cheese roll. Cheeky Charlie grabbed the cheese roll and chewed it. Charlie nearly choked on the cheese roll. Leaving the remains of the cheese roll, Charlie took another child's chips. Next Charlie climbed a cherry tree and chose some ripe cherries to chew. Cheeky Charlie chuckled as he threw some of the cherries down on the children's heads. The children watched as the chimpanzee climbed down the cherry tree. Charlie then chased some chickens across the field. However, Charlie did not look where he was going, and he charged straight into the cheetah's cage. The cheetah jumped up, thrust his muzzle through the bars and bit Charlie on the chin. The chimpanzee howled and ran to Mr Chester. Mr Chester put Cheeky Charlie back into his cage.

Puzzle worksheet for the 'ch' sound

Suitable for children in Years 1 and 2

Use the 'ch' pictures to help you with these puzzles.

Unscramble the words below. They all begin with 'ch'.

1 hspic   **2** klahc   **3** hhccru   **4** hsielc   **5** rryhec

_____   _____   _____   _____   _____

Look for the 'ch' words in the wordsearch below. They can read down or across. There are eight 'ch' words of three letters or more.

c	h	e	r	r	y	a	s
h	d	f	g	j	k	l	z
a	c	h	i	m	n	e	y
i	h	x	c	h	i	n	c
r	a	c	v	b	n	g	h
j	i	c	h	i	c	k	e
l	n	m	x	w	q	b	e
c	h	e	e	s	e	z	k

Write down the words that you found:

1 _____   2 _____

3 _____   4 _____

5 _____   6 _____

7 _____   8 _____

Illustrations for the 'ch' sound

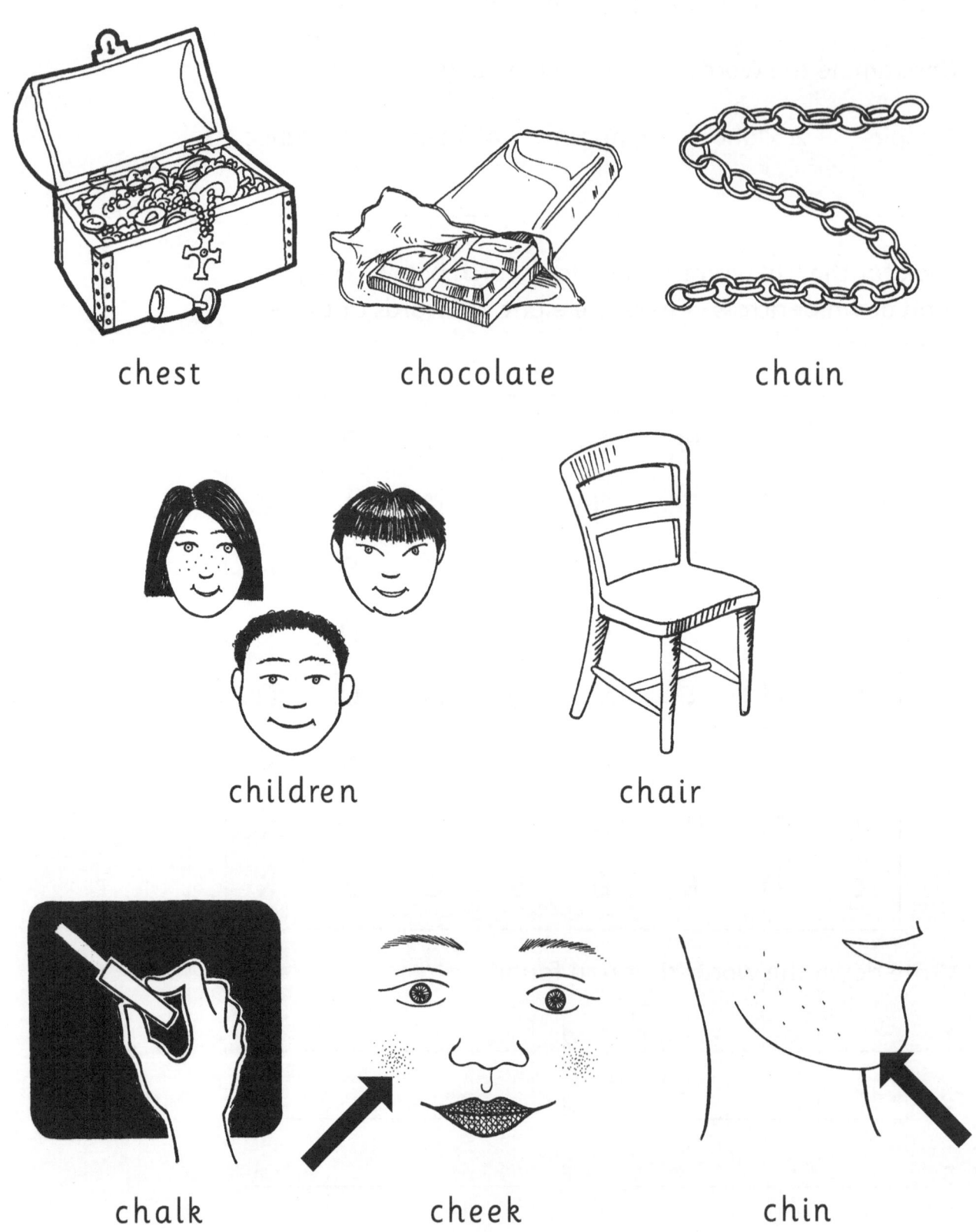

chest

chocolate

chain

children

chair

chalk

cheek

chin

Illustrations for the 'ch' sound

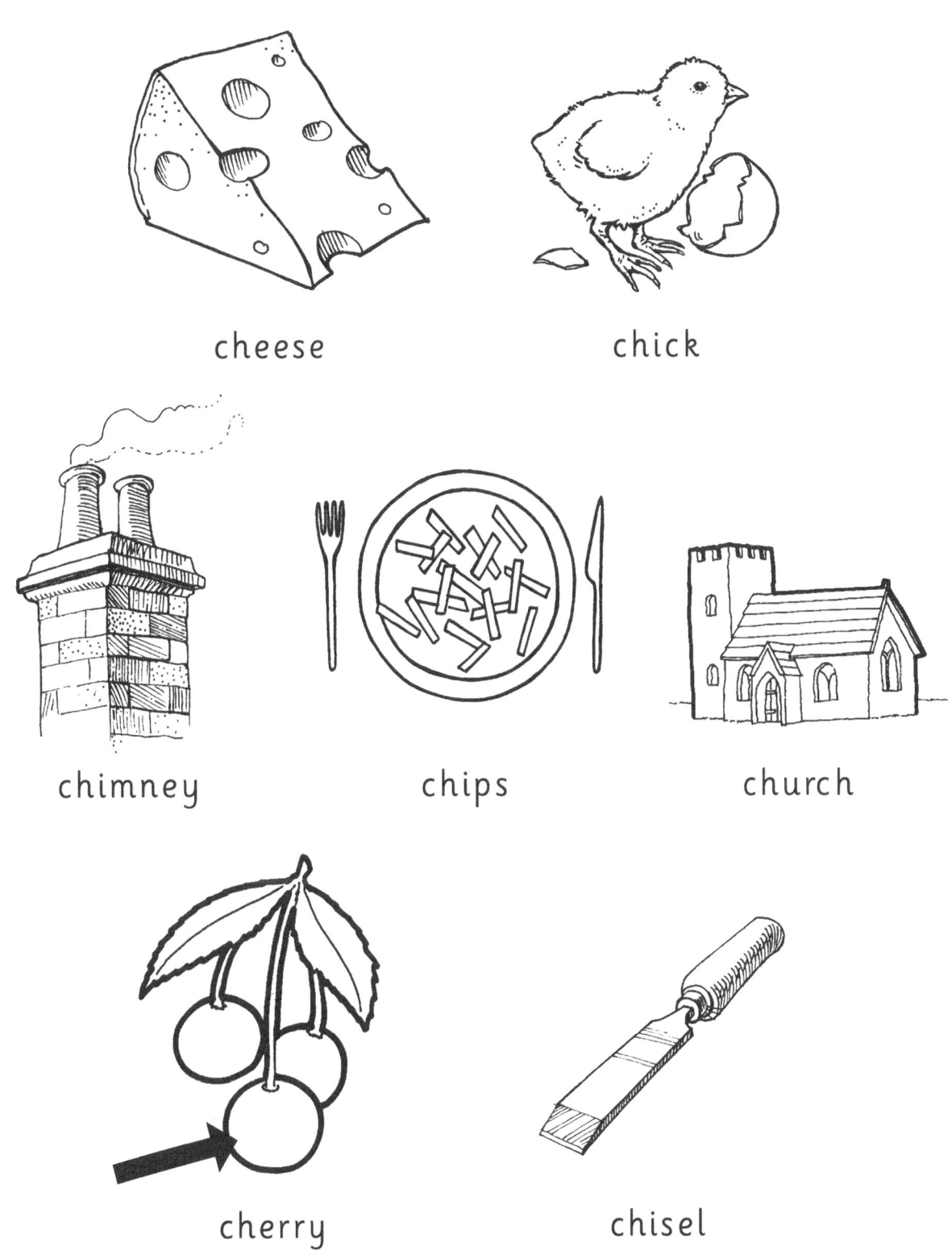

cheese

chick

chimney

chips

church

cherry

chisel

2/2

Answers to stories and puzzle worksheets

Please note: answers in the Story sections appear in sentence order.

Section for the 'b' sound

Story

Bobby's – birthday
bicycle – birthday
Bobby – bed
baby – brother – Bobby
Bobby – birthday – bounced – bed
boxes – bed
Billy – bulldozer
Beth – boat – Bella – book – badgers
Bobby – bicycle
Bobby's – Bobby – back
Bobby – back – back
blue – bicycle – balloons
balloons – Birthday – Bobby

Puzzle worksheet

1 bag **2** bed **3** boat **4** bear **5** bath

| bag | ball | banana | beak |
| bear | bed | boat | bone |

Section for the 'c/k' sound

Story

Callum – Chloe – Cardiff
castle – Candy
Chloe – coconut
coloured – coconuts – could
Callum – candyfloss – covered
cold – Callum – Chloe – car
coats – combed
cooked – cake – cake – cup – coffee
cat – climbed – Callum's
carrot
crawled – Callum – cat – carrot
cat – cry
cat – Callum's – coffee – carpet

Puzzle worksheet

1 cot **2** cat **3** coat **4** cage **5** clock

| cage | cake | camel | coat |
| cobweb | comb | cot | cow |

Section for the 'd' sound

Story

Daniel – Dinah
Daniel – donkey – Dilly – Dinah – duck – Duke
Dougal – dog – dopey
day – Dilly – donkey – Daniel – dinner
Daniel – damaged – Dilly
Daniel – donkey – danger
Dinah – Daniel – Duke – duck
Dilly – Duke
Daniel – donkey – duck
duck – donkey's
donkey – dirty – ditch – daisies – daffodils
doctor – dad
Daniel – doctor – drag – donkey – ditch

Puzzle worksheet

1 dog **2** doll **3** dice **4** duck **5** deer

| daisy | dinner | dinosaur | doll |
| donkey | door | dress | duck |

Section for the 'f' sound

Story

freezing – foggy
Filip – Finlay
fourteen – farm
Filip – Finlay – fields – farm
full – freezing – fog
find – Ferry's – field
find – feel – fence
find – fence – follow

Filip – Finlay – feel
father
Filip – Finlay – father
frightened – freezing – fog
Filip – fuzzy – fog
fox
Finlay – fox – father's – Friday
Filip – Finlay – fox – farmyard
follow – fox – farm
Filip – Finlay – father – find – fox – fled

Puzzle worksheet

1 fan **2** fly **3** four **4** fork **5** fish

face	fan	feather	fin
fish	fly	fork	four

Section for the 'g' sound

Story

Grace – Gabbie – Gilpin – ghost – Guy's
girls – gowns – gloves
green – glowed
granny – gave
getting – ghost
girls – graveyard – Guy's
Grace – Gabbie – gate – gloomy – graveyard
girls – group – ground
grinning
grins – gazed – ghastly – ghosts
gave – great
galloped – gravestones – gap
Grace – Gabbie – grinned
group – grey – Grace's – green – glasses

Puzzle worksheet

1 goat **2** gate **3** girl **4** goose **5** glove

game	garden	gate	ghost
goal	goat	grapes	guitar

Section for the 'h' sound

Story

Heidi – happy – holiday – Heather –
    Heather's
Heather's – house – hotel
Heidi – Heather – helped – heavy – hotel

handle – Heidi's
hopped – Hamish – Heidi's – hamster
Heidi – how – hamster – had
Heidi – Heather – hurried – Hamish – him
hamper – Heather's
hamster – Heather's – hamper
holes – hamper – Hamish
Heidi – hid – hamper – hangers – huge
hamster – happily – hamper – hotel
Hamish – hungry – Heidi – ham – him
holiday – Heidi – her – hamster – her
Heather's – holes – her – hamper – Heather –
    Heidi – her

Puzzle worksheet

1 hat **2** hen **3** hand **4** horse
5 hammer

hair	hand	hat	head
heel	hen	horse	hospital

Section for the 'j' sound

Story

January – Jake – Jill
Jolly – jockey
Jellybeans
Jake – Jill – Jolly – jumpers – jackets – jeans –
    journey
jam
Jake – Jill – jug – juice
Jill – Jake – Jolly
Jolly – Jellybeans
Jill – Jellybeans – jump
jockeys
Jake – Jill – jumped
Jellybeans – jumped – Joker
Jellybeans – Joker
Jellybeans – just – Joker
Jake – Jill – Jolly – jumped – joy

Puzzle worksheet

1 jug **2** jaw **3** jelly **4** jockey **5** jumper

jam	jaw	jelly	jet
jockey	jug	juggler	juice

Section for the 'l' sound

Story

Lucy – Leon – lamb – Lucky
Lucky – leg – lame
Lucy – Leon – Lucky's
Leon – letter
Leon – lazy – like
Lucy – lunch
Lucky – leaping – lame – leg
Lucy – lay – long
look
loud –Lucy
Lucy – lime
lightning – lime – log – leaning – Lucy
Leon – late – Lucy – long
Leon – look – Lucy
Leon – Lucky – loudly
Leon
Looking – lashing – Lucy
Lucy's – leg – log
Leon – lifted – log – Lucy's – leg
Lifted – Lucy – Lucky – leading

Puzzle worksheet

1 leg **2** log **3** lamp **4** lion **5** lemon

ladder   ladybird   lamp   lettuce
lid   lion   lips   log

Section for the 'm' sound

Story

Megan – mischievous – monkey – Mickey
Megan – make – melon – mousse
Mickey – mat – merrily – munching –
    mangoes – marmalade
Megan – melon
melon – mixing – mixed
Megan – mate – Martha
meet – Martha
Meanwhile – mischievous – monkey – melon
    – mixture
marched – mustard – making – mess
Megan – mess
mischievous – monkey – mashed – milk

Puzzle worksheet

1 mop **2** mug **3** milk **4** meat
5 money

man   map   money   monkey
moon   mountain   mouse   mug

Section for the 'n' sound

Story

Noah – newspaper
needed – new
Noah – ninety
Noah – nice – new – newspapers
Noah – noticed
knee – knuckles – nose
Noah – knelt – necklace
Noah – Nelson
notice – not
Noah – knocked – Nelson
necklace
Noah – necklace
Nicola – nurse – number – nineteen
nephew – Nathan – necklace
Noah – nine – notes
Nicola – knee – knuckles – nose

Puzzle worksheet

1 nut **2** neck **3** nail **4** nurse **5** needle

nail   neck   needle   nest
net   nine   nose   nurse

Section for the 'p' sound

Story

Pedro's – post – purchase
post – Pedro – passage – park
park – Pedro – passed – people
passed – pony – pale – pet – parrot
parrot – pecking – pocket
Pedro – paused – perched – park
PAINT
Pedro – people – playing – pond
Pedro – purple – pink
proceeded – post – purchased
Pedro – park – passage
Pedro's – pleased – purchased – pleased – pink
    – purple

Puzzle worksheet

1 pen **2** pig **3** pear **4** panda
5 pepper

paint	panda	parrot	pear
pen	pig	plate	pond

Section for the 'r' sound

Story

Ruby – road – river – rain
rats – ran – road – Ruby
Ruby – run
raining – Ruby – raincoat
red – ring – rolled – river
Ruby – remembered – Ria
ran – Ria's – Regent – Road – rang
Ria – Ruby – ring
Ruby – Ria – river
Ria – reeds
ringing
Ria – rested – rock
ran – rough – reeds
rubbish – ring
Ria – Ruby – ring – returned
reaching – Ruby – raincoat
red – ring – raincoat

Puzzle worksheet

1 ram **2** rain **3** rope **4** river **5** rocket

rabbit	rainbow	rat	ribbon
ring	road	rocket	rug

Section for the 's' sound

Story

summer's – sun
Sydney – sister – Sophie – sea
So – Sydney – Sophie – sun – swimsuits – sat – sand
Sydney – sandcastle – Sophie – sand
sausages – salmon – sandwiches – salt
strawberry – six – sweet
Sydney – Sophie – sandals – sea
sisters – stood – stared – sea
saw – surfboard

Suddenly – surfboarder – swept – surfboard
surfboarder – seemed – struggling – swim
Sydney – sister
said – surfboarder
swam – surfboarder – saved
surfboarder – sisters – sense

Puzzle worksheet

1 six **2** salt **3** sink **4** soup **5** sausage

saddle	salt	scissors	seven
sink	six	soap	sock

Section for the 't' sound

Story

Tuesday – Toby – Tyler – Todd
Todd – town – twenty
To – to – take – to – train
trip – took – two
Toby – Tyler – Tennyson – twelve
twelve – Tennyson – trees
Toby – Tyler – terrible
Todd – tuba
Toby – Tyler – touched
Todd's – Timothy – to
told – Todd – today – tidied – toys
Toby – Tyler – to – talk – to – Todd
Toby – Tyler – to – Todd – to – tidy – toys
Todd's – told – to – time – telephoned
Toby – Tyler – turned – two – Tollbridge

Puzzle worksheet

1 tent **2** table **3** tiger **4** teeth
5 tomato

tail	tap	tea	ten
tie	toast	tortoise	two

Section for the 'v' and 'w' sounds

Stories

The 'v' sound
Victoria
Virgil – vet's
violin – vicar
Victoria – visited – Venus

Victoria – Venus – village
Venus' – Vinny – van
Vinny – van – Vauxhall – Victoria – Venus
Venus – velvet – Val's
Victoria – vests – vase
Venus – vanilla
Victoria – Venus – Vanessa
very
Victoria – Venus – Vauxhall – Vinny – van –
 vanished
Victoria – Venus – very – Venus'

The 'w' sound
Wayne – watch
Wilf – was
Wayne – Wilf – were – watch
Wolverhampton – Wanderers – were –
 Wallsend – Willow
Wayne – walk – Willow
wet – windy – Wayne – wore – Wellington –
 warm
Wayne – walked – Water – Wicker
Wayne's – wet
Willow – Wayne
waterlogged – will – Wednesday
wet – Wayne – walked – Wilf's
Willis – Wilf – wet – walking – work
Willis – wanted – wake – Wilf
Willis – wet – Wayne – was – warm
Willis – Wayne's – wet – washing
Wayne – Wilf's – walk

Puzzle worksheet
1 van **2** vest **3** witch **4** water
5 watch

van	vase	vest	violin
wall	window	wing	witch

Section for the 'y' and 'th' sounds

Stories
The 'y' sound
Yasmin – young – Yummy – yo-yos
Yasmin – yo-yo – Yummy
Yummy – yelped – yellow
yolks

Yummy – yolks
Yasmin – yelled – Yummy
Yummy – yacht
Yasmin – yellow
Yasmin
Yasmin – year
Yasmin – yellow – Yummy – yogurt

The 'th' (unvoiced) sound
Theo – Thornton – Thackery – throwing –
 thrush
thrush – through – thick
three – through – thrush
Theo – thumb – thorn – throbbed
Thackery – throat – thistle – Thornton –
 thigh
Thrower – thrush
three – throwing – things
Thrower – thick – thrush
Thankfully – thirty – thrush
three – thunderstorm
Theo – Thackery – Thornton – thunder
three – Thrower's – thunder
three – Thrower's
Theo – Thackery – Thornton – thrushes'
three – three – thrushes
thrashed – throw – thrushes
three – throw – thrushes
Theo – Thackery – Thornton – thrush

Puzzle worksheet
1 yawn **2** yolk **3** thumb **4** thorn
5 three

thorn	thread	three	throat
thumb	yacht	yawn	yolk

Section for the 'sh' sound

Story
Sherry – shower – shampooed
she – shirt – shorts – shoes
she – shutting
short – Shore
she – shop – shortcake – Shane – share
Shane – she
Shane – shelves – Sharp's – Shelton

Sherry – shivering – shelter – Shadwell – Shelton

Sherry – Shelton – short – sharp – shower

shorts – shins

Sherry – shaking – she

She – shut

she – Shane – shouting

She – shoulder – Shane

showed – Sherry

shut – short

Shane's – shiny – Sharp's

Sherry – shelter – Shadwell

Puzzle worksheet

1 shark **2** shirt **3** shelf **4** shorts
5 shell

shampoo	shed	sheep	shelf
shell	ship	shoe	shop

Section for the 'ch' sound

Story

Cheeky – Charlie – chimpanzee

Chester – Charlie's – Charlie

child – cheese

Cheeky – Charlie – cheese – chewed

Charlie – choked – cheese

cheese – Charlie – child's – chips

Charlie – cherry – chose – cherries – chew

Cheeky – Charlie – chuckled – cherries – children's

children – chimpanzee – cherry

Charlie – chased – chickens

Charlie – charged – cheetah's

cheetah – Charlie – chin

chimpanzee – Chester

Chester – Cheeky – Charlie

Puzzle worksheet

1 chips **2** chalk **3** church **4** chisel
5 cherry

chain	chair	cheek	cheese
cherry	chick	chimney	chin

194